ROYAL JELLY

A MEDICAL DICTIONARY, BIBLIOGRAPHY,
AND ANNOTATED RESEARCH GUIDE TO
INTERNET REFERENCES

JAMES N. PARKER, M.D.
AND PHILIP M. PARKER, PH.D., EDITORS

ICON Health Publications
ICON Group International, Inc.
4370 La Jolla Village Drive, 4th Floor
San Diego, CA 92122 USA

Printed in the United States of America.

Last digit indicates print number: 10 9 8 7 6 4 5 3 2 1

Publisher, Health Care: Philip Parker, Ph.D.
Editor(s): James Parker, M.D., Philip Parker, Ph.D.

Publisher's note: The ideas, procedures, and suggestions contained in this book are not intended for the diagnosis or treatment of a health problem. As new medical or scientific information becomes available from academic and clinical research, recommended treatments and drug therapies may undergo changes. The authors, editors, and publisher have attempted to make the information in this book up to date and accurate in accord with accepted standards at the time of publication. The authors, editors, and publisher are not responsible for errors or omissions or for consequences from application of the book, and make no warranty, expressed or implied, in regard to the contents of this book. Any practice described in this book should be applied by the reader in accordance with professional standards of care used in regard to the unique circumstances that may apply in each situation. The reader is advised to always check product information (package inserts) for changes and new information regarding dosage and contraindications before prescribing any drug or pharmacological product. Caution is especially urged when using new or infrequently ordered drugs, herbal remedies, vitamins and supplements, alternative therapies, complementary therapies and medicines, and integrative medical treatments.

Cataloging-in-Publication Data

Parker, James N., 1961-
Parker, Philip M., 1960-

    Royal Jelly: A Medical Dictionary, Bibliography, and Annotated Research Guide to Internet References / James N. Parker and Philip M. Parker, editors
               p.   cm.
    Includes bibliographical references, glossary, and index.
    ISBN: 0-597-84297-3
    1. Royal Jelly-Popular works.   I. Title.

Disclaimer

This publication is not intended to be used for the diagnosis or treatment of a health problem. It is sold with the understanding that the publisher, editors, and authors are not engaging in the rendering of medical, psychological, financial, legal, or other professional services.

References to any entity, product, service, or source of information that may be contained in this publication should not be considered an endorsement, either direct or implied, by the publisher, editors, or authors. ICON Group International, Inc., the editors, and the authors are not responsible for the content of any Web pages or publications referenced in this publication.

Copyright Notice

Acknowledgements

The collective knowledge generated from academic and applied research summarized in various references has been critical in the creation of this book which is best viewed as a comprehensive compilation and collection of information prepared by various official agencies which produce publications on royal jelly. Books in this series draw from various agencies and institutions associated with the United States Department of Health and Human Services, and in particular, the Office of the Secretary of Health and Human Services (OS), the Administration for Children and Families (ACF), the Administration on Aging (AOA), the Agency for Healthcare Research and Quality (AHRQ), the Agency for Toxic Substances and Disease Registry (ATSDR), the Centers for Disease Control and Prevention (CDC), the Food and Drug Administration (FDA), the Healthcare Financing Administration (HCFA), the Health Resources and Services Administration (HRSA), the Indian Health Service (IHS), the institutions of the National Institutes of Health (NIH), the Program Support Center (PSC), and the Substance Abuse and Mental Health Services Administration (SAMHSA). In addition to these sources, information gathered from the National Library of Medicine, the United States Patent Office, the European Union, and their related organizations has been invaluable in the creation of this book. Some of the work represented was financially supported by the Research and Development Committee at INSEAD. This support is gratefully acknowledged. Finally, special thanks are owed to Tiffany Freeman for her excellent editorial support.

About the Editors

James N. Parker, M.D.

Dr. James N. Parker received his Bachelor of Science degree in Psychobiology from the University of California, Riverside and his M.D. from the University of California, San Diego. In addition to authoring numerous research publications, he has lectured at various academic institutions. Dr. Parker is the medical editor for health books by ICON Health Publications.

Philip M. Parker, Ph.D.

Philip M. Parker is the Eli Lilly Chair Professor of Innovation, Business and Society at INSEAD (Fontainebleau, France and Singapore). Dr. Parker has also been Professor at the University of California, San Diego and has taught courses at Harvard University, the Hong Kong University of Science and Technology, the Massachusetts Institute of Technology, Stanford University, and UCLA. Dr. Parker is the associate editor for ICON Health Publications.

About ICON Health Publications

To discover more about ICON Health Publications, simply check with your preferred online booksellers, including Barnes&Noble.com and Amazon.com which currently carry all of our titles. Or, feel free to contact us directly for bulk purchases or institutional discounts:

ICON Group International, Inc.
4370 La Jolla Village Drive, Fourth Floor
San Diego, CA 92122 USA
Fax: 858-546-4341
Web site: **www.icongrouponline.com/health**

Table of Contents

FORWARD

In March 2001, the National Institutes of Health issued the following warning: "The number of Web sites offering health-related resources grows every day. Many sites provide valuable information, while others may have information that is unreliable or misleading."[1] Furthermore, because of the rapid increase in Internet-based information, many hours can be wasted searching, selecting, and printing. Since only the smallest fraction of information dealing with royal jelly is indexed in search engines, such as **www.google.com** or others, a non-systematic approach to Internet research can be not only time consuming, but also incomplete. This book was created for medical professionals, students, and members of the general public who want to know as much as possible about royal jelly, using the most advanced research tools available and spending the least amount of time doing so.

In addition to offering a structured and comprehensive bibliography, the pages that follow will tell you where and how to find reliable information covering virtually all topics related to royal jelly, from the essentials to the most advanced areas of research. Public, academic, government, and peer-reviewed research studies are emphasized. Various abstracts are reproduced to give you some of the latest official information available to date on royal jelly. Abundant guidance is given on how to obtain free-of-charge primary research results via the Internet. **While this book focuses on the field of medicine, when some sources provide access to non-medical information relating to royal jelly, these are noted in the text.**

E-book and electronic versions of this book are fully interactive with each of the Internet sites mentioned (clicking on a hyperlink automatically opens your browser to the site indicated). If you are using the hard copy version of this book, you can access a cited Web site by typing the provided Web address directly into your Internet browser. You may find it useful to refer to synonyms or related terms when accessing these Internet databases. **NOTE:** At the time of publication, the Web addresses were functional. However, some links may fail due to URL address changes, which is a common occurrence on the Internet.

For readers unfamiliar with the Internet, detailed instructions are offered on how to access electronic resources. For readers unfamiliar with medical terminology, a comprehensive glossary is provided. For readers without access to Internet resources, a directory of medical libraries, that have or can locate references cited here, is given. We hope these resources will prove useful to the widest possible audience seeking information on royal jelly.

The Editors

---

[1] From the NIH, National Cancer Institute (NCI): **http://www.cancer.gov/cancerinfo/ten-things-to-know**.

CHAPTER 1. STUDIES ON ROYAL JELLY

Overview

In this chapter, we will show you how to locate peer-reviewed references and studies on royal jelly.

Federally Funded Research on Royal Jelly

The U.S. Government supports a variety of research studies relating to royal jelly. These studies are tracked by the Office of Extramural Research at the National Institutes of Health.[2] CRISP (Computerized Retrieval of Information on Scientific Projects) is a searchable database of federally funded biomedical research projects conducted at universities, hospitals, and other institutions.

Search the CRISP Web site at **http://crisp.cit.nih.gov/crisp/crisp_query.generate_screen**. You will have the option to perform targeted searches by various criteria, including geography, date, and topics related to royal jelly.

For most of the studies, the agencies reporting into CRISP provide summaries or abstracts. As opposed to clinical trial research using patients, many federally funded studies use animals or simulated models to explore royal jelly.

The National Library of Medicine: PubMed

One of the quickest and most comprehensive ways to find academic studies in both English and other languages is to use PubMed, maintained by the National Library of Medicine.[3]

---

[2] Healthcare projects are funded by the National Institutes of Health (NIH), Substance Abuse and Mental Health Services (SAMHSA), Health Resources and Services Administration (HRSA), Food and Drug Administration (FDA), Centers for Disease Control and Prevention (CDCP), Agency for Healthcare Research and Quality (AHRQ), and Office of Assistant Secretary of Health (OASH).

[3] PubMed was developed by the National Center for Biotechnology Information (NCBI) at the National Library of Medicine (NLM) at the National Institutes of Health (NIH). The PubMed database was developed in conjunction with publishers of biomedical literature as a search tool for accessing literature citations and linking to full-text

The advantage of PubMed over previously mentioned sources is that it covers a greater number of domestic and foreign references. It is also free to use. If the publisher has a Web site that offers full text of its journals, PubMed will provide links to that site, as well as to sites offering other related data. User registration, a subscription fee, or some other type of fee may be required to access the full text of articles in some journals.

To generate your own bibliography of studies dealing with royal jelly, simply go to the PubMed Web site at **http://www.ncbi.nlm.nih.gov/pubmed**. Type "royal jelly" (or synonyms) into the search box, and click "Go." The following is the type of output you can expect from PubMed for royal jelly (hyperlinks lead to article summaries):

- **Allergic reactions to honey and royal jelly and their relationship with sensitization to compositae.**
  Author(s): Lombardi C, Senna GE, Gatti B, Feligioni M, Riva G, Bonadonna P, Dama AR, Canonica GW, Passalacqua G.
  Source: Allergologia Et Immunopathologia. 1998 November-December; 26(6): 288-90.
  http://www.ncbi.nlm.nih.gov:80/entrez/query.fcgi?cmd=Retrieve&db=PubMed&list_uids=9934408&dopt=Abstract

- **Allergies to wheat, yeast and royal jelly: a connection between ingestion and inhalation?**
  Author(s): Baldo BA.
  Source: Monogr Allergy. 1996; 32: 84-91. Review. No Abstract Available.
  http://www.ncbi.nlm.nih.gov:80/entrez/query.fcgi?cmd=Retrieve&db=PubMed&list_uids=8813187&dopt=Abstract

- **Asthma and anaphylaxis induced by royal jelly.**
  Author(s): Thien FC, Leung R, Baldo BA, Weiner JA, Plomley R, Czarny D.
  Source: Clinical and Experimental Allergy : Journal of the British Society for Allergy and Clinical Immunology. 1996 February; 26(2): 216-22.
  http://www.ncbi.nlm.nih.gov:80/entrez/query.fcgi?cmd=Retrieve&db=PubMed&list_uids=8835130&dopt=Abstract

- **Asthma following royal jelly.**
  Author(s): Harwood M, Harding S, Beasley R, Frankish PD.
  Source: N Z Med J. 1996 August 23; 109(1028): 325. No Abstract Available.
  http://www.ncbi.nlm.nih.gov:80/entrez/query.fcgi?cmd=Retrieve&db=PubMed&list_uids=8816730&dopt=Abstract

- **Bronchospasm induced by royal jelly.**
  Author(s): Laporte JR, Ibaanez L, Vendrell L, Ballarin E.
  Source: Allergy. 1996 June; 51(6): 440.
  http://www.ncbi.nlm.nih.gov:80/entrez/query.fcgi?cmd=Retrieve&db=PubMed&list_uids=8837671&dopt=Abstract

journal articles at Web sites of participating publishers. Publishers that participate in PubMed supply NLM with their citations electronically prior to or at the time of publication.

- **Case report: haemorrhagic colitis associated with royal jelly intake.**
  Author(s): Yonei Y, Shibagaki K, Tsukada N, Nagasu N, Inagaki Y, Miyamoto K, Suzuki O, Kiryu Y.
  Source: Journal of Gastroenterology and Hepatology. 1997 July; 12(7): 495-9.
  http://www.ncbi.nlm.nih.gov:80/entrez/query.fcgi?cmd=Retrieve&db=PubMed&list_uids=9257239&dopt=Abstract

- **Contact dermatitis due to honeybee royal jelly.**
  Author(s): Takahashi M, Matsuo I, Ohkido M.
  Source: Contact Dermatitis. 1983 November; 9(6): 452-5.
  http://www.ncbi.nlm.nih.gov:80/entrez/query.fcgi?cmd=Retrieve&db=PubMed&list_uids=6653102&dopt=Abstract

- **Effect of royal jelly on mitotic activity of lymphocytes.**
  Author(s): Vittek J, Tajmirova O.
  Source: Biologia (Bratisl). 1968; 23(9): 699-702. No Abstract Available.
  http://www.ncbi.nlm.nih.gov:80/entrez/query.fcgi?cmd=Retrieve&db=PubMed&list_uids=5681907&dopt=Abstract

- **Effect of royal jelly on serum lipids in experimental animals and humans with atherosclerosis.**
  Author(s): Vittek J.
  Source: Experientia. 1995 September 29; 51(9-10): 927-35. Review.
  http://www.ncbi.nlm.nih.gov:80/entrez/query.fcgi?cmd=Retrieve&db=PubMed&list_uids=7556573&dopt=Abstract

- **Fatal royal jelly-induced asthma.**
  Author(s): Bullock RJ, Rohan A, Straatmans JA.
  Source: The Medical Journal of Australia. 1994 January 3; 160(1): 44.
  http://www.ncbi.nlm.nih.gov:80/entrez/query.fcgi?cmd=Retrieve&db=PubMed&list_uids=8271989&dopt=Abstract

- **N-linked sugar chains of 350-kDa royal jelly glycoprotein.**
  Author(s): Kimura Y, Washino N, Yonekura M.
  Source: Bioscience, Biotechnology, and Biochemistry. 1995 March; 59(3): 507-9.
  http://www.ncbi.nlm.nih.gov:80/entrez/query.fcgi?cmd=Retrieve&db=PubMed&list_uids=7766191&dopt=Abstract

- **Respiratory distress and royal jelly.**
  Author(s): Peacock S, Murray V, Turton C.
  Source: Bmj (Clinical Research Ed.). 1995 December 2; 311(7018): 1472.
  http://www.ncbi.nlm.nih.gov:80/entrez/query.fcgi?cmd=Retrieve&db=PubMed&list_uids=8520337&dopt=Abstract

- **Royal jelly consumption and hypersensitivity in the community.**
  Author(s): Leung R, Ho A, Chan J, Choy D, Lai CK.
  Source: Clinical and Experimental Allergy : Journal of the British Society for Allergy and Clinical Immunology. 1997 March; 27(3): 333-6.
  http://www.ncbi.nlm.nih.gov:80/entrez/query.fcgi?cmd=Retrieve&db=PubMed&list_uids=9088660&dopt=Abstract

- **Royal jelly-induced asthma and anaphylaxis: clinical characteristics and immunologic correlations.**
  Author(s): Leung R, Thien FC, Baldo B, Czarny D.
  Source: The Journal of Allergy and Clinical Immunology. 1995 December; 96(6 Pt 1): 1004-7.
  http://www.ncbi.nlm.nih.gov:80/entrez/query.fcgi?cmd=Retrieve&db=PubMed&list_uids=8543734&dopt=Abstract

- **Royal jelly-induced asthma.**
  Author(s): Thien FC, Leung R, Plomley R, Weiner J, Czarny D.
  Source: The Medical Journal of Australia. 1993 November 1; 159(9): 639.
  http://www.ncbi.nlm.nih.gov:80/entrez/query.fcgi?cmd=Retrieve&db=PubMed&list_uids=8123114&dopt=Abstract

CHAPTER 2. NUTRITION AND ROYAL JELLY

Overview

In this chapter, we will show you how to find studies dedicated specifically to nutrition and royal jelly.

Finding Nutrition Studies on Royal Jelly

The National Institutes of Health's Office of Dietary Supplements (ODS) offers a searchable bibliographic database called the IBIDS (International Bibliographic Information on Dietary Supplements; National Institutes of Health, Building 31, Room 1B29, 31 Center Drive, MSC 2086, Bethesda, Maryland 20892-2086, Tel: 301-435-2920, Fax: 301-480-1845, E-mail: ods@nih.gov). The IBIDS contains over 460,000 scientific citations and summaries about dietary supplements and nutrition as well as references to published international, scientific literature on dietary supplements such as vitamins, minerals, and botanicals.[4] The IBIDS includes references and citations to both human and animal research studies.

As a service of the ODS, access to the IBIDS database is available free of charge at the following Web address: **http://ods.od.nih.gov/databases/ibids.html**. After entering the search area, you have three choices: (1) IBIDS Consumer Database, (2) Full IBIDS Database, or (3) Peer Reviewed Citations Only.

Now that you have selected a database, click on the "Advanced" tab. An advanced search allows you to retrieve up to 100 fully explained references in a comprehensive format. Type "royal jelly" (or synonyms) into the search box, and click "Go." To narrow the search, you can also select the "Title" field.

---

[4] Adapted from **http://ods.od.nih.gov**. IBIDS is produced by the Office of Dietary Supplements (ODS) at the National Institutes of Health to assist the public, healthcare providers, educators, and researchers in locating credible, scientific information on dietary supplements. IBIDS was developed and will be maintained through an interagency partnership with the Food and Nutrition Information Center of the National Agricultural Library, U.S. Department of Agriculture.

The following information is typical of that found when using the "Full IBIDS Database" to search for "royal jelly" (or a synonym):

- **A family of major royal jelly proteins of the honeybee Apis mellifera L.**
  Author(s): Laboratory of Genetic Engineering, Slovak Academy of Sciences, Bratislava, Slovakia. chemjakl@savba.sk
  Source: Schmitzova, J Klaudiny, J Albert, S Schroder, W Schreckengost, W Hanes, J Judova, J Simuth, J Cell-Mol-Life-Sci. 1998 September; 54(9): 1020-30 1420-682X

- **A potent antibacterial protein in royal jelly. Purification and determination of the primary structure of royalisin.**
  Author(s): Biochemical Research Laboratory, Morinaga Milk Industry Company Limited, Kanagawa, Japan.
  Source: Fujiwara, S Imai, J Fujiwara, M Yaeshima, T Kawashima, T Kobayashi, K J-Biol-Chem. 1990 July 5; 265(19): 11333-7 0021-9258

- **A royal jelly as a new potential immunomodulator in rats and mice.**
  Author(s): Department of Biology, University of Zagreb, Croatia.
  Source: Sver, L Orsolic, N Tadic, Z Njari, B Valpotic, I Basic, I Comp-Immunol-Microbiol-Infect-Dis. 1996 January; 19(1): 31-8 0147-9571

- **A royal jelly protein is expressed in a subset of Kenyon cells in the mushroom bodies of the honey bee brain.**
  Author(s): Research School of Biological Sciences, Australian National University, Canberra, Australia.
  Source: Kucharski, R Maleszka, R Hayward, D C Ball, E E Naturwissenschaften. 1998 July; 85(7): 343-6 0028-1042

- **Allergic reactions to honey and royal jelly and their relationship with sensitization to compositae.**
  Author(s): Dept. of Internal Medicine Sant'Orsola Hospital, Brescia, Italy.
  Source: Lombardi, C Senna, G E Gatti, B Feligioni, M Riva, G Bonadonna, P Dama, A R Canonica, G W Passalacqua, G Allergol-Immunopathol-(Madr). 1998 Nov-December; 26(6): 288-90 0301-0546

- **Allergies to wheat, yeast and royal jelly: a connection between ingestion and inhalation?**
  Author(s): Kolling Institute of Medical Research, Royal North Shore Hospital of Sydney, St Leonards, N.S.W., Australia.
  Source: Baldo, B A Monogr-Allergy. 1996; 3284-91 0077-0760

- **Analysis of Drosophila yellow-B cDNA reveals a new family of proteins related to the royal jelly proteins in the honeybee and to an orphan protein in an unusual bacterium Deinococcus radiodurans.**
  Author(s): Visual Sciences, Research School of Biological Sciences, Canberra, ACT, 0200, Australia. maleszka@rsbs.anu.edu.au
  Source: Maleszka, R Kucharski, R Biochem-Biophys-Res-Commun. 2000 April 21; 270(3): 773-6 0006-291X

- **Antifatigue effect of fresh royal jelly in mice.**
  Author(s): POLA R&D Laboratories, POLA Corporation, Yokohama, Japan. m-kamakura@pola.co.jp
  Source: Kamakura, M Mitani, N Fukuda, T Fukushima, M J-Nutr-Sci-Vitaminol-(Tokyo). 2001 December; 47(6): 394-401 0301-4800

- **Antimicrobial potency of royal jelly collected from queen cells at different larvae ages.**
  Author(s): Cairo Univ., Fayoum (Egypt). Faculty of Agriculture
  Source: Abd Alla, M.S. Mishrei, A. Ghazi, I.M. Annals-of-Agricultural-Science (Egypt). (December 1995). volume 40(2) page 597-608. Issued 1996. royal jelly apis mellifera larvae bacteria mortality antimicrobial properties

- **Apisimin, a new serine-valine-rich peptide from honeybee (Apis mellifera L.) royal jelly: purification and molecular characterization.**
  Author(s): Laboratory of Genetic Engineering, Institute of Chemistry, Slovak Academy of Sciences, Dubravska cesta 9, SK-84238 Bratislava, Slovak Republic.
  Source: Bilikova, K Hanes, J Nordhoff, E Saenger, W Klaudiny, J Simuth, J FEBS-Lett. 2002 September 25; 528(1-3): 125-9 0014-5793

- **Application of solid/liquid extraction for the gravimetric determination of lipids in royal jelly.**
  Author(s): French Food Safety Agency (AFSSA), Unite Abeille, B.P. 111, F-06902 Sophia Antipolis Cedex, France. jf.antinelli@sophia.afssa.fr
  Source: Antinelli, Jean Francois Davico, Renee Rognone, Catherine Faucon, Jean Paul Lizzani Cuvelier, Louisette J-Agric-Food-Chem. 2002 April 10; 50(8): 2227-30 0021-8561

- **Asthma and anaphylaxis induced by royal jelly.**
  Author(s): Department of Respiratory Medicine, Alfred Hospital, Prahran, Australia.
  Source: Thien, F C Leung, R Baldo, B A Weiner, J A Plomley, R Czarny, D Clin-Exp-Allergy. 1996 February; 26(2): 216-22 0954-7894

- **Augmentation of wound healing by royal jelly (RJ) in streptozotocin-diabetic rats.**
  Author(s): Department of Pharmacology, Nihon University School of Dentistry, Matsudo, Japan.
  Source: Fujii, A Kobayashi, S Kuboyama, N Furukawa, Y Kaneko, Y Ishihama, S Yamamoto, H Tamura, T Jpn-J-Pharmacol. 1990 July; 53(3): 331-7 0021-5198

- **Bronchospasm induced by royal jelly.**
  Author(s): Institut Catala de Farmacologia, Universitat Autonoma de Barcelona, Spain.
  Source: Laporte, J R Ibaanez, L Vendrell, L Ballarin, E Allergy. 1996 June; 51(6): 440 0105-4538

- **Case report: haemorrhagic colitis associated with royal jelly intake.**
  Author(s): Department of Internal Medicine, Nippon Kokan Hospital, Kanagawa, Japan.
  Source: Yonei, Y Shibagaki, K Tsukada, N Nagasu, N Inagaki, Y Miyamoto, K Suzuki, O Kiryu, Y J-Gastroenterol-Hepatol. 1997 July; 12(7): 495-9 0815-9319

- **Determination and confirmation of methyl p-hydroxybenzoate in royal jelly and other foods produced by the honey bee.**
  Author(s): National Institute of Health Sciences, Tokyo, Japan.
  Source: Ishiwata, H Takeda, Y Yamada, T Watanabe, Y Hosagai, T Ito, S Sakurai, H Aoki, G Ushiama, N Food-Addit-Contam. 1995 Mar-April; 12(2): 281-5 0265-203X

- **Determination of trans-10-hydroxy-2-decenoic acid content in pure royal jelly and royal jelly products by column liquid chromatography.**
  Author(s): Ege University, Engineering Faculty, Food Engineering Department, Bornova-Izmir, Turkey. genc@textil.eg.edu.tr
  Source: Genc, M Aslan, A J-Chromatogr-A. 1999 April 16; 839(1-2): 265-8

- **Effect of royal jelly on guinea-pig growth.**
  Source: Afifi, E.A. Khattab, M.M. El Berry, A.A. Abdel Gawaad, A.A. Proceedings of the Fourth International Conference on Apiculture in Tropical Climates, Cairo, Egypt, 6-10

November 1988 / hosted by the government of Egypt; convened by the International Bee Research Association. London : International Bee Research Association, 1989. page 42-45. ISBN: 0860981967

- **Fifty-seven-kDa protein in royal jelly enhances proliferation of primary cultured rat hepatocytes and increases albumin production in the absence of serum.**
  Author(s): POLA R&D Laboratories, POLA Corporation, 560 Kashio-cho, Totuka-ku, Yokohama, 244-0812, Japan. m-kamakura@pola.co.jp
  Source: Kamakura, M Suenobu, N Fukushima, M Biochem-Biophys-Res-Commun. 2001 April 13; 282(4): 865-74 0006-291X

- **Furosine: a suitable marker for assessing the freshness of royal jelly.**
  Author(s): DISTAAM, Universita del Molise, Via De Sanctis, 86100 Campobasso, Italy. marconi@unimol.it
  Source: Marconi, Emanuele Caboni, Maria Fiorenza Messia, Maria Cristina Panfili, Gianfranco J-Agric-Food-Chem. 2002 May 8; 50(10): 2825-9 0021-8561

- **Growth stimulation with honey royal jelly DIII protein of human lymphocytic cell lines in a serum-free medium.**
  Author(s): School of Agriculture, Ibaraki University, 3-21-1 Ami, Ibaraki 300-03 (Japan)
  Source: Watanabe, K. Shinmoto, H. Kobori, M. Tsushida, T. Shinohara, K. Kanaeda, J. Yonekura, M. Biotechnology-Techniques (United Kingdom). (1996). volume 10(12) page 959-962. honeycomb extracts lymphocytes mankind royal jelly proteins

- **Inhibition of specific degradation of 57-kDa protein in royal jelly during storage by ethylenediaminetetraacetic acid.**
  Author(s): POLA R&D Laboratories, POLA Corporation, Yokohama, Japan. m-kamakura@pola.co.jp
  Source: Kamakura, M Fukushima, M Biosci-Biotechnol-Biochem. 2002 January; 66(1): 175-8 0916-8451

- **Isolation of a peptide fraction from honeybee royal jelly as a potential antifoolbrood factor.**
  Author(s): Slovak Academy of Sciences, Bratislava (Slovaquie). Institute of Chemistry, Laboratory of Genetic Engineering
  Source: Bilikova, K. Wu, G. Simuth, J. Apidologie (France). (Mai-June 2001). volume 32(3) page 275-283. apis mellifera royal jelly peptides antibiotic properties foul brood bacillus larvae 0044-8435

- **Liquid chromatographic determination of trans-10-hydroxy-2-decenoic acid content of commercial products containing royal jelly.**
  Author(s): Institute of Science and Forensic Medicine, Singapore.
  Source: Bloodworth, B C Harn, C S Hock, C T Boon, Y O J-AOAC-Int. 1995 Jul-August; 78(4): 1019-23 1060-3271

- **Molecular characterization of MRJP3, highly polymorphic protein of honeybee (Apis mellifera) royal jelly.**
  Author(s): Laboratory of Genetic Engineering, Slovak Academy of Sciences, Bratislava, Slovak Republic. salbert@gwdg.de
  Source: Albert, S Klaudiny, J Simuth, J Insect-Biochem-Mol-Biol. 1999 May; 29(5): 427-34 0965-1748

- **N-linked sugar chain of 55-kDa royal jelly glycoprotein.**
  Author(s): Department of Bioresources Chemistry, Faculty of Agriculture, Okayama University, Japan.

Source: Kimura, Y Kajiyama, S Kanaeda, J Izukawa, T Yonekura, M Biosci-Biotechnol-Biochem. 1996 December; 60(12): 2099-102 0916-8451

- **Oxytetracycline residues in honey and royal jelly.**
  Source: Matsuka, M. Nakamura, J. J-Apic-Res. London : International Bee Research Association. 1990. volume 29 (2) page 112-117. 0021-8839

- **Physiological effect of royal jelly on female reproductive capacity in rabbits.**
  Source: Khattab, M.M. Radwan, A.A. Afifi, E.A. Proceedings of the Fourth International Conference on Apiculture in Tropical Climates, Cairo, Egypt, 6-10 November 1988 / hosted by the government of Egypt; convened by the International Bee Research Association. London : International Bee Research Association, 1989. page 70-73. ISBN: 0860981967

- **Preparation of recombinant most abundant protein MRJP1 of royal jelly.**
  Author(s): Slovak Academy of Sciences, Bratislava (Slovak Republic). Institute of Chemistry
  Source: Judova, J. Klaudiny, J. Simuth, J. Biologia (Slovak Republic). Section Cellular and Molecular Biology. (1998). volume 53(6) page 777-784. honeybees royal jelly proteins hypersensitivity 0006-3088

- **Reproductive responses following royal jelly treatment administered orally or intramuscularly into progesterone-treated Awassi ewes.**
  Author(s): Department of Animal Production, Faculty of Agriculture, Jordan University of Science and Technology, PO Box 3030, 22110, Irbid, Jordan. huseinmq@just.edu.jo
  Source: Husein, M Q Kridli, R T Anim-Reprod-Sci. 2002 November 15; 74(1-2): 45-53 0378-4320

- **Respiratory distress and royal jelly.**
  Author(s): Royal Sussex County Hospital, Brighton.
  Source: Peacock, S Murray, V Turton, C BMJ. 1995 December 2; 311(7018): 1472 0959-8138

- **Royal jelly in apitherapy [Diet and disease, nutritive value for humans]. Laptisorul de matca in apiterapie.**
  Source: Anastasiu, R.I. Apicultura. Bucuresti, Romania : Ministerul Agriculturil, Industriei Alimentare si Apelor. July 1982. volume 57 (7) page 22. 0378-2425

- **Royal jelly: mystery food. 2.**
  Source: Iannuzzi, J. Am-Bee-J. Hamilton, Ill. : Dadant & Sons. Sept 1990. volume 130 (9) page 587-589. 0002-7626

- **Signal Transduction Mechanism Leading to Enhanced Proliferation of Primary Cultured Adult Rat Hepatocytes Treated with Royal Jelly 57-kDa Protein.**
  Author(s): POLA R&D Laboratories, POLA Corporation, Kashio-cho, Totuka-ku, Yokohama 244-0812, Japan. m-kamakura@pop16.odn.ne.jp
  Source: Kamakura, M J-Biochem-(Tokyo). 2002 December; 132(6): 911-9 0021-924X

- **Storage-dependent degradation of 57-kDa protein in royal jelly: a possible marker for freshness.**
  Author(s): POLA R&D Laboratories, POLA Corporation, Yokohama, Japan. m-kamakura@pola.co.jp
  Source: Kamakura, M Fukuda, T Fukushima, M Yonekura, M Biosci-Biotechnol-Biochem. 2001 February; 65(2): 277-84 0916-8451

- **Structural features of N-glycans linked to royal jelly glycoproteins: structures of high-mannose type, hybrid type, and biantennary type glycans.**
  Author(s): Department of Bioresources Chemistry, Faculty of Agriculture, Okayama University, Japan. yosh8mar@cc.okayama-u.ac.jp
  Source: Kimura, Y Miyagi, C Kimura, M Nitoda, T Kawai, N Sugimoto, H Biosci-Biotechnol-Biochem. 2000 October; 64(10): 2109-20 0916-8451

- **Suppression of allergic reactions by royal jelly in association with the restoration of macrophage function and the improvement of Th1/Th2 cell responses.**
  Author(s): Central Research Laboratories, Zeria Pharmaceutical Co., Ltd., 2512-1 Oshikiri, Kohnan-machi, Ohsato-gun, Saitama 360-0111, Japan.
  Source: Oka, H Emori, Y Kobayashi, N Hayashi, Y Nomoto, K Int-Immunopharmacol. 2001 March; 1(3): 521-32 1567-5769

- **The effect of soluble sugars in stored royal jelly on the differentiation of female honeybee (Apis mellifera L.) larvae to queens.**
  Source: Asencot, M. Lensky, Y. Insect-Biochem. Oxford : Pergamon Press. 1988. volume 18 (2) page 127-133. ill. 0020-1790

- **The family of major royal jelly proteins and its evolution.**
  Author(s): Laboratory of Genetic Engineering, Institute of Chemistry, Slovak Academy of Sciences, Dubravska cesta 9, SK-842 38 Bratislava, Slovakia.
  Source: Albert, S Bhattacharya, D Klaudiny, J Schmitzova, J Simuth, J J-Mol-Evol. 1999 August; 49(2): 290-7 0022-2844

Federal Resources on Nutrition

In addition to the IBIDS, the United States Department of Health and Human Services (HHS) and the United States Department of Agriculture (USDA) provide many sources of information on general nutrition and health. Recommended resources include:

- healthfinder®, HHS's gateway to health information, including diet and nutrition: **http://www.healthfinder.gov/scripts/SearchContext.asp?topic=238&page=0**

- The United States Department of Agriculture's Web site dedicated to nutrition information: **www.nutrition.gov**

- The Food and Drug Administration's Web site for federal food safety information: **www.foodsafety.gov**

- The National Action Plan on Overweight and Obesity sponsored by the United States Surgeon General: **http://www.surgeongeneral.gov/topics/obesity/**

- The Center for Food Safety and Applied Nutrition has an Internet site sponsored by the Food and Drug Administration and the Department of Health and Human Services: **http://vm.cfsan.fda.gov/**

- Center for Nutrition Policy and Promotion sponsored by the United States Department of Agriculture: **http://www.usda.gov/cnpp/**

- Food and Nutrition Information Center, National Agricultural Library sponsored by the United States Department of Agriculture: **http://www.nal.usda.gov/fnic/**

- Food and Nutrition Service sponsored by the United States Department of Agriculture: **http://www.fns.usda.gov/fns/**

Additional Web Resources

A number of additional Web sites offer encyclopedic information covering food and nutrition. The following is a representative sample:

- AOL: **http://search.aol.com/cat.adp?id=174&layer=&from=subcats**

- Family Village: **http://www.familyvillage.wisc.edu/med_nutrition.html**

- Google: **http://directory.google.com/Top/Health/Nutrition/**

- Healthnotes: **http://www.healthnotes.com/**

- Open Directory Project: **http://dmoz.org/Health/Nutrition/**

- Yahoo.com: **http://dir.yahoo.com/Health/Nutrition/**

- WebMD®Health: **http://my.webmd.com/nutrition**

- WholeHealthMD.com: **http://www.wholehealthmd.com/reflib/0,1529,00.html**

The following is a specific Web list relating to royal jelly; please note that any particular subject below may indicate either a therapeutic use, or a contraindication (potential danger), and does not reflect an official recommendation:

- **Food and Diet**

     High Cholesterol
     Source: Healthnotes, Inc.; www.healthnotes.com

Chapter 3. Alternative Medicine and Royal Jelly

Overview

In this chapter, we will begin by introducing you to official information sources on complementary and alternative medicine (CAM) relating to royal jelly. At the conclusion of this chapter, we will provide additional sources.

National Center for Complementary and Alternative Medicine

The National Center for Complementary and Alternative Medicine (NCCAM) of the National Institutes of Health (**http://nccam.nih.gov/**) has created a link to the National Library of Medicine's databases to facilitate research for articles that specifically relate to royal jelly and complementary medicine. To search the database, go to the following Web site: **http://www.nlm.nih.gov/nccam/camonpubmed.html**. Select "CAM on PubMed." Enter "royal jelly" (or synonyms) into the search box. Click "Go." The following references provide information on particular aspects of complementary and alternative medicine that are related to royal jelly:

- **Antifatigue effect of fresh royal jelly in mice.**
  Author(s): Kamakura M, Mitani N, Fukuda T, Fukushima M.
  Source: J Nutr Sci Vitaminol (Tokyo). 2001 December; 47(6): 394-401.
  http://www.ncbi.nlm.nih.gov:80/entrez/query.fcgi?cmd=Retrieve&db=PubMed&list_uids=11922114&dopt=Abstract

- **Bee health and international trade.**
  Author(s): Shimanuki H, Knox DA.
  Source: Rev Sci Tech. 1997 April; 16(1): 172-6. Review.
  http://www.ncbi.nlm.nih.gov:80/entrez/query.fcgi?cmd=Retrieve&db=PubMed&list_uids=9329115&dopt=Abstract

- **Bioactive natural compounds for the treatment of gastrointestinal disorders.**
  Author(s): Ghosh S, Playford RJ.

Source: Clinical Science (London, England : 1979). 2003 June; 104(6): 547-56. Review.
http://www.ncbi.nlm.nih.gov:80/entrez/query.fcgi?cmd=Retrieve&db=PubMed&list_
uids=12641494&dopt=Abstract

- **Change in the expression of hypopharyngeal-gland proteins of the worker honeybees (Apis mellifera L.) with age and/or role.**
  Author(s): Kubo T, Sasaki M, Nakamura J, Sasagawa H, Ohashi K, Takeuchi H, Natori S.
  Source: Journal of Biochemistry. 1996 February; 119(2): 291-5.
  http://www.ncbi.nlm.nih.gov:80/entrez/query.fcgi?cmd=Retrieve&db=PubMed&list_
  uids=8882720&dopt=Abstract

- **Complementary and alternative medicine in children with asthma.**
  Author(s): Orhan F, Sekerel BE, Kocabas CN, Sackesen C, Adalioglu G, Tuncer A.
  Source: Annals of Allergy, Asthma & Immunology : Official Publication of the American College of Allergy, Asthma, & Immunology. 2003 June; 90(6): 611-5.
  http://www.ncbi.nlm.nih.gov:80/entrez/query.fcgi?cmd=Retrieve&db=PubMed&list_
  uids=12839318&dopt=Abstract

- **Contact dermatitis due to honeybee royal jelly.**
  Author(s): Takahashi M, Matsuo I, Ohkido M.
  Source: Contact Dermatitis. 1983 November; 9(6): 452-5.
  http://www.ncbi.nlm.nih.gov:80/entrez/query.fcgi?cmd=Retrieve&db=PubMed&list_
  uids=6653102&dopt=Abstract

- **Determination and confirmation of methyl p-hydroxybenzoate in royal jelly and other foods produced by the honey bee.**
  Author(s): Ishiwata H, Takeda Y, Yamada T, Watanabe Y, Hosagai T, Ito S, Sakurai H, Aoki G, Ushiama N.
  Source: Food Additives and Contaminants. 1995 March-April; 12(2): 281-5.
  http://www.ncbi.nlm.nih.gov:80/entrez/query.fcgi?cmd=Retrieve&db=PubMed&list_
  uids=7781824&dopt=Abstract

- **Disposition of ampicillin in honeybees and hives.**
  Author(s): Nakajima C, Okayama A, Sakogawa T, Nakamura A, Hayama T.
  Source: The Journal of Veterinary Medical Science / the Japanese Society of Veterinary Science. 1997 September; 59(9): 765-7.
  http://www.ncbi.nlm.nih.gov:80/entrez/query.fcgi?cmd=Retrieve&db=PubMed&list_
  uids=9342699&dopt=Abstract

- **Disposition of mirosamicin in honeybee hives.**
  Author(s): Nakajima C, Sakogawa T, Okayama A, Nakamura A, Hayama T.
  Source: Journal of Veterinary Pharmacology and Therapeutics. 1998 August; 21(4): 269-73.
  http://www.ncbi.nlm.nih.gov:80/entrez/query.fcgi?cmd=Retrieve&db=PubMed&list_
  uids=9731948&dopt=Abstract

- **Diverse biological activities of healthy foods.**
  Author(s): Kobayashi N, Unten S, Kakuta H, Komatsu N, Fujimaki M, Satoh K, Aratsu C, Nakashima H, Kikuchi H, Ochiai K, Sakagami H.

Source: In Vivo. 2001 January-February; 15(1): 17-23.
http://www.ncbi.nlm.nih.gov:80/entrez/query.fcgi?cmd=Retrieve&db=PubMed&list_
uids=11286123&dopt=Abstract

- **Immunological aspects of Chinese medicinal plants as antiageing drugs.**
  Author(s): Xiao PG, Xing ST, Wang LW.
  Source: Journal of Ethnopharmacology. 1993 March; 38(2-3): 167-75. Review.
  http://www.ncbi.nlm.nih.gov:80/entrez/query.fcgi?cmd=Retrieve&db=PubMed&list_
  uids=8510465&dopt=Abstract

- **Inhibition of specific degradation of 57-kDa protein in royal jelly during storage by ethylenediaminetetraacetic acid.**
  Author(s): Kamakura M, Fukushima M.
  Source: Bioscience, Biotechnology, and Biochemistry. 2002 January; 66(1): 175-8.
  http://www.ncbi.nlm.nih.gov:80/entrez/query.fcgi?cmd=Retrieve&db=PubMed&list_
  uids=11866102&dopt=Abstract

- **Research in the field of antiviral chemotherapy performed in the "Stefan S. Nicolau" Institute of Virology.**
  Author(s): Esanu V.
  Source: Virologie. 1984 October-December; 35(4): 281-93.
  http://www.ncbi.nlm.nih.gov:80/entrez/query.fcgi?cmd=Retrieve&db=PubMed&list_
  uids=6097022&dopt=Abstract

- **Royal Jelly prolongs the life span of C3H/HeJ mice: correlation with reduced DNA damage.**
  Author(s): Inoue S, Koya-Miyata S, Ushio S, Iwaki K, Ikeda M, Kurimoto M.
  Source: Experimental Gerontology. 2003 September; 38(9): 965-9.
  http://www.ncbi.nlm.nih.gov:80/entrez/query.fcgi?cmd=Retrieve&db=PubMed&list_
  uids=12954483&dopt=Abstract

- **Signal transduction mechanism leading to enhanced proliferation of primary cultured adult rat hepatocytes treated with royal jelly 57-kDa protein.**
  Author(s): Kamakura M.
  Source: Journal of Biochemistry. 2002 December; 132(6): 911-9.
  http://www.ncbi.nlm.nih.gov:80/entrez/query.fcgi?cmd=Retrieve&db=PubMed&list_
  uids=12473193&dopt=Abstract

- **Social exploitation of vitellogenin.**
  Author(s): Amdam GV, Norberg K, Hagen A, Omholt SW.
  Source: Proceedings of the National Academy of Sciences of the United States of America. 2003 February 18; 100(4): 1799-802. Epub 2003 Feb 03.
  http://www.ncbi.nlm.nih.gov:80/entrez/query.fcgi?cmd=Retrieve&db=PubMed&list_
  uids=12566563&dopt=Abstract

- **Traditional remedies and food supplements. A 5-year toxicological study (1991-1995).**
  Author(s): Shaw D, Leon C, Kolev S, Murray V.

Source: Drug Safety : an International Journal of Medical Toxicology and Drug Experience. 1997 November; 17(5): 342-56.
http://www.ncbi.nlm.nih.gov:80/entrez/query.fcgi?cmd=Retrieve&db=PubMed&list_uids=9391777&dopt=Abstract

- **Unproven diet therapies in the treatment of the chronic fatigue syndrome.**
  Author(s): Morris DH, Stare FJ.
  Source: Archives of Family Medicine. 1993 February; 2(2): 181-6. Review.
  http://www.ncbi.nlm.nih.gov:80/entrez/query.fcgi?cmd=Retrieve&db=PubMed&list_uids=8275187&dopt=Abstract

Additional Web Resources

A number of additional Web sites offer encyclopedic information covering CAM and related topics. The following is a representative sample:

- Alternative Medicine Foundation, Inc.: **http://www.herbmed.org/**

- AOL: **http://search.aol.com/cat.adp?id=169&layer=&from=subcats**

- Chinese Medicine: **http://www.newcenturynutrition.com/**

- drkoop.com®: **http://www.drkoop.com/InteractiveMedicine/IndexC.html**

- Family Village: **http://www.familyvillage.wisc.edu/med_altn.htm**

- Google: **http://directory.google.com/Top/Health/Alternative/**

- Healthnotes: **http://www.healthnotes.com/**

- MedWebPlus:
  http://medwebplus.com/subject/Alternative_and_Complementary_Medicine

- Open Directory Project: **http://dmoz.org/Health/Alternative/**

- HealthGate: **http://www.tnp.com/**

- WebMD®Health: **http://my.webmd.com/drugs_and_herbs**

- WholeHealthMD.com: **http://www.wholehealthmd.com/reflib/0,1529,00.html**

- Yahoo.com: **http://dir.yahoo.com/Health/Alternative_Medicine/**

The following is a specific Web list relating to royal jelly; please note that any particular subject below may indicate either a therapeutic use, or a contraindication (potential danger), and does not reflect an official recommendation:

- **Alternative Therapy**

    Apitherapy
    Source: WholeHealthMD.com, LLC.; www.wholehealthmd.com
    Hyperlink:
    http://www.wholehealthmd.com/refshelf/substances_view/0,1525,669,00.html

- **Herbs and Supplements**

  Bee Products
  Source: WholeHealthMD.com, LLC.; www.wholehealthmd.com
  Hyperlink:
  http://www.wholehealthmd.com/refshelf/substances_view/0,1525,756,00.html

  Pollen
  Source: Healthnotes, Inc.; www.healthnotes.com

  Royal Jelly
  Source: Healthnotes, Inc.; www.healthnotes.com

General References

A good place to find general background information on CAM is the National Library of Medicine. It has prepared within the MEDLINEplus system an information topic page dedicated to complementary and alternative medicine. To access this page, go to the MEDLINEplus site at **http://www.nlm.nih.gov/medlineplus/alternativemedicine.html**. This Web site provides a general overview of various topics and can lead to a number of general sources.

CHAPTER 4. PATENTS ON ROYAL JELLY

Overview

Patents can be physical innovations (e.g. chemicals, pharmaceuticals, medical equipment) or processes (e.g. treatments or diagnostic procedures). The United States Patent and Trademark Office defines a patent as a grant of a property right to the inventor, issued by the Patent and Trademark Office.[5] Patents, therefore, are intellectual property. For the United States, the term of a new patent is 20 years from the date when the patent application was filed. If the inventor wishes to receive economic benefits, it is likely that the invention will become commercially available within 20 years of the initial filing. It is important to understand, therefore, that an inventor's patent does not indicate that a product or service is or will be commercially available. The patent implies only that the inventor has "the right to exclude others from making, using, offering for sale, or selling" the invention in the United States. While this relates to U.S. patents, similar rules govern foreign patents.

In this chapter, we show you how to locate information on patents and their inventors. If you find a patent that is particularly interesting to you, contact the inventor or the assignee for further information. **IMPORTANT NOTE:** When following the search strategy described below, you may discover <u>non-medical patents</u> that use the generic term "royal jelly" (or a synonym) in their titles. To accurately reflect the results that you might find while conducting research on royal jelly, <u>we have not necessarily excluded non-medical patents</u> in this bibliography.

Patents on Royal Jelly

By performing a patent search focusing on royal jelly, you can obtain information such as the title of the invention, the names of the inventor(s), the assignee(s) or the company that owns or controls the patent, a short abstract that summarizes the patent, and a few excerpts from the description of the patent. The abstract of a patent tends to be more technical in nature, while the description is often written for the public. Full patent descriptions contain much more information than is presented here (e.g. claims, references, figures, diagrams, etc.). We will tell you how to obtain this information later in the chapter. The following is an

---

[5]Adapted from the United States Patent and Trademark Office:
http://www.uspto.gov/web/offices/pac/doc/general/whatis.htm.

example of the type of information that you can expect to obtain from a patent search on royal jelly:

- **Breast-enhancing, herbal compositions and methods of using same**

  Inventor(s): Ernest; Joseph Michael (Oceanside, CA), Smith; Allen (Encino, CA)

  Assignee(s): Vital Dynamics, Inc. (canoga Park, Ca)

  Patent Number: 6,200,594

  Date filed: December 29, 1999

  Abstract: Topical and oral compositions containing unique blends of certain herbs effectively enhance breasts in human females by strengthening connective tissues and encouraging the growth of new cells. The topical composition contains Saw Palmetto berry extract, Chaste Tree berry extract, Fenugreek seed extract, Fennel seed extract, Comfrey extract, White Willow Bark extract, Ma Huang extract, Black Cohosh extract, Guarana extract, Passion Flower extract, Bilberry extract, Horsetail extract and Cayenne extract. The oral composition is a dietary supplement system containing two diet supplement compositions. The first composition contains extracts of Blessed Thistle, Hops, Wild Yam, Fenugreek seed, Saw Palmetto berry, Chaste Tree berry, Fennel seed, Black Cohosh, Damiana, Dong Quai, Lycium Chinese Herb, Scullcap Concentrate, and Curcubita Pepo Pumpkin seed, as well as Methyl Sulfonyl Methane and **Royal Jelly.** The second composition contains extracts of Saw Palmetto berry, Chaste Tree berry, Black Cohosh, Fennel seed, Fenugreek seed, Lycium Chinese Herb, Scullcap Concentrate, and Curcubita Pepo Pumpkin seed, as well as Methyl Sulfonyl Methane and **Royal Jelly.** The topical composition, which is preferably in cream form, is topically applied to the breast area daily for a sufficient period of time. The oral system, preferably in the form of a plurality of capsules taken separately, is orally administered on a daily basis for a sufficient period, wherein capsules of the first composition are taken for a first period and capsules of the second composition are taken for a subsequent second period. Most preferably, the topical and oral compositions are administered concurrently in a treatment regimen. The latter regimen provides a synergistic breast enhancement relative to the individual topical and oral treatments.

  Excerpt(s): The present invention relates to compositions and methods for enhancing breasts. More particularly, this invention relates to herbal topical and oral compositions and methods of using same to enhance breast appearance in women. An attractive bustline is important to many women. Unfortunately, as women age, lose weight or become inactive, their bustlines tend to become less firm and, therefore, less attractive. The strengthening or building up of biological tissue in the female human breast is a well known problem in physiotherapy. One medical approach uses surgical techniques, such as breast implant operations. Such approach has numerous disadvantages. For example, surgical operations are inherently dangerous and relatively expensive. Opting for use of a surgical breast implant carries with it not only the danger and expense involved in any surgical operation but also potential health dangers that may be associated with using a particular type of breast implant, namely, the silicone breast implant.

  Web site: http://www.delphion.com/details?pn=US06200594__

- **Extractor for recovering royal jelly from artificial honeycomb lathes**

  Inventor(s): Horr; Bohumir Z. (306 W. 93rd St., New York, NY 10025)

  Assignee(s): None Reported

  Patent Number: 5,326,304

  Date filed: June 1, 1993

  Abstract: A rotationally-driven piston used as an extractor for recovering bee's **royal jelly** in the use of which a mixture of lavre and **royal jelly** is expelled by centrifugal force against a lavre-removal screen which results in only the **royal jelly** continuing therethrough to a surrounding piston chamber wall, from which the **royal jelly** is then scraped during manual movement of a piston head axially of the piston chamber.

  Excerpt(s): This invention relates to the collection and recovery of honey, and more particularly to queen's **royal jelly,** using artificial honeycombs and the use of centrifugal force. It is already well known that plural lathes with a lengthwise arrangement of cups thereon which comprise the artificial honeycomb can be removed from a bee hive super, placed in a centrifuge, and using centrifugal force have the honey contents of the cups expelled therefrom. In accordance with the specific objects of the present invention, the cups are more particularly queen's cups, and the recovery is of **royal jelly** from the fluid **royal jelly** and particulate lavre contents of the queen's cups. The methodology of achieving filled queen's cups of a mixture of fluid **royal jelly** and particulate lavre on removable lathes preparatory to the harvesting of the **royal jelly** component of the mixture is, as already noted, well known in the patent literature, as exemplified by U.S. Pat. No. 3,840,925 issued on Oct. 15, 1974 to Kenneth F. Croan for "Method of Recovering Honey from Artificial Honeycombs" and U.S. Pat. No. 1,791,605 issued on Feb. 10, 1931 to H. H. Root entitled "Radial Extractor and Method of Extracting Honey". The operating mode of the aforesaid, and all other similar devices using centrifugal force, has significant shortcomings when applied to the collection and recovery of queen's **royal jelly,** due primarily to the highly viscous nature of this fluid which renders it inappropriate to rely on its gravity flow from the centrifuge, and which heretofore has been an unsatisfactorily solved obstacle.

  Web site: http://www.delphion.com/details?pn=US05326304__

- **Frame assembly for collecting royal jelly**

  Inventor(s): Hong; Keum P. (Av. Amores 1126, Dep. 201, Colonia del Valle, MX), Hong; Soon Y. (Av. Amores 1126, Dep. 201, Colonia del Valle, MX)

  Assignee(s): None Reported

  Patent Number: 4,672,704

  Date filed: November 21, 1985

  Abstract: A molded plastic frame, especially for collecting **royal jelly,** is disclosed. The frame includes a horizontal top frame member which has at each one of its respective ends formations for engaging and locking, with the engaging formations including a tapering surface formation, and the locking formations include a locking lip. The frame also has at least two vertically disposable side member assemblies which can be releasably connected to the top frame member in such a way that they are releasably connected by way of an insert mode which precludes the removal of a respective side member without deformation of the locking lip. The frame assembly also includes at least one transverse jelly cup bar which can be connected to the frame between the vertically disposed side members assemblies.

Excerpt(s): The invention may be classified in class 6 and appropriate sub-classes. Our present invention relates generally to improvements in or relating to apiarian frames and, more particularly, to an improved frame assembly which is comprised of individual interconnectable frame components made of molded plastic. Still more particularly, our invention relates to a molded plastic frame assembly comprised of individual components, which frame serves to collect **royal jelly.**

Web site: http://www.delphion.com/details?pn=US04672704__

- **Herbal hormone balance composition**

Inventor(s): Chun; Zhang (1665 E. Fourth St., #109, Santa Ana, CA 92701)

Assignee(s): None Reported

Patent Number: 6,238,707

Date filed: October 11, 2000

Abstract: The present invention comprises a selection of herbal, organic and inorganic materials with curative effects combined in a powdered form for human ingestion. The demonstrated benefits on human female hormone regulation or replacement include return from irregular to regular and less painful menstrual cycles, raising estrogen and progesterone levels to normal levels through menstrual cycles, return to regular menstrual cycle hormone levels with apparent infertility cure, and return to normative metabolic response from apparent circulatory abnormalities such as excessive sweating, edema, cold hand and feet, stiffness and other such symptoms. The hormone regulation powder comprises motherwort, Epimedium (barrenwort), Polygonum multiforum root and stem (fleece flower), millettia stem, Paeoniae radix (red Peony root), Achyranthes bidentata, Albizia julibrissin, Philodendron domesticum, Lycium barbarum, oyster shell, cow placenta, **royal jelly,** vitamin E, Astragalus chinensis and Gardenia augusta or jasminoides and further optionally comprises Wolfberry fruit, ginseng, asia bell, chinese angelica root, Rehmannia glutinosa, donkey hide gelatin, white peony root, Poris cocos, chinese yam or piloce antler.

Excerpt(s): The present invention relates to herbal compositions for female human hormone replacement or regulation. Lycium chinense (Cortex of Wolfberry root) and Gardenia jasminoides have been found to be of importance as a component of an herbal composition in U.S. Pat. No. 5,874,084 for hot flashes (intense heat sensation, flushing, profuse sweating, palpitations, and/or sense of anxiety) stating that such occurrences for a menopausal woman may be substantially eliminated or ameliorated by administering to a woman in need of treatment an effective amount of ingestible material which has as substantially the only active ingredient a herbal complex. Motherwort is described as a component in a topical paste in U.S. Pat. No. 5,968,518 comprising as active ingredients chickweed, yarrow, wormwood, motherwort, pennyroyal, and dandelion in a vehicle of olive-oil and beeswax.

Web site: http://www.delphion.com/details?pn=US06238707__

- **Method and apparatus for the harvesting of royal jelly**

  Inventor(s): Fraser-Jones; Anthony Paul (Bethell, NZ)

  Assignee(s): Royal Jelly New Zealand Limited (waitakere, Nz)

  Patent Number: 5,830,039

  Date filed: March 18, 1997

  Abstract: A method and apparatus for the harvesting of **royal jelly**. The method comprises the use of a first matrix of cell-like structures in an arrangement typical of normal worker bee cells which have interconnected plugs placed in the back of the matrix. A queen bee may then lay this matrix of cells with eggs. Upon the eggs turning into larvae, the plugs may be removed and the plugs are provided in interconnected sets such that each set provides plugs for each alternate cell in the first matrix of cells. These plugs may then be fitted to a second matrix of cells which provide larger, queen-like cells at a spacing of substantially the same as the alternate cells in the first matrix. The second matrix may then be placed in a queenless hive for the bees to fill the larger cells of the second matrix with **royal jelly** which may then be harvested.

  Excerpt(s): This invention relates to methods and apparatus for the harvesting of **royal jelly** and, in particular, a method and apparatus related to the use of interchangeable artificial cells for the collection of **royal jelly**. Royal jelly is a natural product produced by bees in a hive to feed larvae and queen bees. All larvae in the hive receive a quantity of **royal jelly** for sustenance in their early stages. Subsequently, the **royal jelly** is withheld from all but queen bees. Therefore, although the largest single quantities of **royal jelly** can be found in queen cell hives, the largest quantity of cells receiving **royal jelly** are in fact those of the normal worker bee. On this basis, the normal method of harvesting **royal jelly** is to remove the larvae and the small quantities of **royal jelly** produced into each of the numerous larvae cells from these cells. Each of these small quantities of **royal jelly** may be removed from the worker bee cell and placed into a much larger cell which would normally house the larva for a queen bee. When this larger cell is placed into a queenless hive, the bees will concentrate on filling this queen cell with **royal jelly** for the production of a queen bee.

  Web site: http://www.delphion.com/details?pn=US05830039__

- **Method for the preparation of powderized honey products, the products obtained according to the method and their use**

  Inventor(s): Schanze; Rudolf (Neumarkt, DE)

  Assignee(s): None Reported

  Patent Number: 4,504,516

  Date filed: February 8, 1983

  Abstract: A powdered honey product containing 50-85% of honey or a mixture of honey and at least one bee product selected from the group consisting of beebread, pollen **royal jelly,** drone syrup, green syrup, beeswax, propolis and propolis extract, 5-25% silica and 25-35% polymeric carbohydrate.

  Excerpt(s): The present invention relates to a method for preparing powdered honey products, to the products obtained by the method and to the use of the powdered bee products. In general, bee products, in particular honey, also drone syrup and queen bee syrup, propolis, propolis extracts (bee glue), which are dissolved in the honey as well as pollen and beebread, which are also distributed in the honey, are extremely viscid-plastic, heavy-flowing viscous materials. In addition to their food value, which can be different depending on the product but which however is always very high, these products are endowed with additional health-promoting, sickness preventing, and in short biological properties. These properties are based on materials contained in the bee products, which in part already derive from the plant food of the bees, however which in the larger part are generated by the working and processing through the bees, and which are enriched in the bee products and which provide these biological properties. (Compare for example Edmund Herold "Health values from the bee colony", 6th edition, 1970, Publisher: Ehrenwirth-Verlag, Munich). The varied and beneficial effects of these materials are known overall. However, the composition of these materials is still not finally known, and some of the materials have not been identified. However, it is established that these materials are extremely sensitive, in particular to heating. Therefore, bee products are in general stored at temperatures in the range of from -15 to +13 degrees centigrade. In the case of honey, it is provided that any crystallization is prevented, since crystallization favors fermentation and thus leads to spoilage. The particular effects of the bee products are in part ascribed to hormone, to enzyme and to vitamin-like groups of active agents, in part to complex mineral trace element groups, of which it is also known that they can be increasingly sensitive to a heating beyond the range of from 35 to 40 degrees centigrade.

Web site: http://www.delphion.com/details?pn=US04504516__

- **Method for the treatment of symptoms related to normal hormonal variations in wome**

  Inventor(s): Hedman; Christer (Molnlycke, SE), Karnerud; Lars (Tenhult, SE), Winther; Kaj (Copenhagen, DK)

  Assignee(s): Natumin Pharma AB (huskvarna, Se)

  Patent Number: 6,569,471

  Date filed: August 31, 2001

  Abstract: A method for the treatment of symptoms related to normal hormonal variations in women during fertile, peri- and post-menopausal age, by the administering of a composition comprising, as active ingredients, a water and/or fat-soluble cytosolic extract of pollen, optionally combined with **Royal Jelly** and Vitamin E.

  Excerpt(s): The invention relates in a first aspect to a method for the treatment of symptoms related to normal hormonal variations in women during fertile as well as, peri- and post-menopausal age, by the administering of a composition comprising, as active ingredients, a water and/or fat soluble cytosolic extract of pollen, optionally combined with **Royal Jelly** and Vitamin E. The invention, in another aspect, relates to the use of a composition comprising, as active ingredients, a water and/or fat soluble extract of pollen optionally combined with **Royal Jelly** and Vitamin E for the manufacturing of a medicament for the treatment of symptoms relating to normal hormonal variations in women during fertile, as well as peri- and post-menopausal age. An extract of combined pollen and pistils combined with a pollen grain extract, **Royal Jelly** and Vitamin E has been sold by Interhealth AB, Kungsangsvagen 27, 561 56 Huskvarna, Sweden, for the treatment of Pre-Menstrual Syndrome (PMS).

  Web site: http://www.delphion.com/details?pn=US06569471__

- **Method for the treatment of symptoms related to normal hormonal variations in wome**

Inventor(s): Hedman; Christer (Molnlycke, SE), Karnerud; Lars (Tenhult, SE), Winter; Kaj (Copenhage, DK)

Assignee(s): Natumin Pharma AB (huskvarna, Se)

Patent Number: 6,669,967

Date filed: June 28, 2002

Abstract: A method for the treatment of disorders related to normal hormonal variations in women during fertile, peri- and post-menopausal age, by the administering of a composition comprising, as active ingredients, a water and/or fat-soluble cytosolic extract of pollen and optionally pistils, optionally combined with **Royal Jelly** and vitamin E.

Excerpt(s): The invention relates in a first aspect to a method for the treatment of disorders related to normal hormonal variations in women during fertile as well as, peri- and post-menopausal age, by the administering of a composition comprising, as active ingredients, a water- and/or fat-soluble cytosolic extract of pollen and optionally pistils. The invention, in another aspect, relates to a composition comprising, as active ingredients, a water- and/or fat-soluble cytosolic extract of pollen and optionally pistils for the treatment of disorders relating to normal hormonal variations in women during fertile, as well as peri- and post-menopausal age. Disorders relating to normal variation of the sex hormone cycle of women of fertile age are tension, irritability, dysphoria, abdominal distension or bloatedness, severe breast tension, headache or migraine, edema, weight changes, sleep disturbances etc. The overall well being as well as the social and professional life may be influenced.

Web site: http://www.delphion.com/details?pn=US06669967__

- **Prepared royal jelly with caloric value**

Inventor(s): Nomura; Masayuki (Kanagawa, JP), Xu; Ying Ying (Kanagawa, JP)

Assignee(s): Cera Rica Noda Co., Ltd. (kanagawa, Jp)

Patent Number: 6,521,274

Date filed: April 4, 2000

Abstract: Provided is a preparative **royal jelly** with low caloric value, which contains a raw **royal jelly,** erythritol and oligosaccharide derived from soybean, and is in the form of a paste.

Excerpt(s): The present invention relates to a preparative **royal jelly** excellent in its taste and human health. The **royal jelly** is a viscous substance with milk-white or pale yellowish color, which is given to honey bee larvae and a queen bee and has been known from old times as efficacious one of perpetual youth and longevity, nourishment, robustness and so on. The **royal jelly** as commodities is classified into a--raw royal jelly---,--dried royal jelly--which is lyophilized product of the raw **royal jelly,** and--preparative royal jelly--which is prepared by composing an auxiliary material or additive to the raw or dried **royal jelly** and has been marketed as a healthy food, alimentary and roborantal preparation or nutriental supplement.

Web site: http://www.delphion.com/details?pn=US06521274__

- **Process for the obtainment of a biologically active bee-product**

  Inventor(s): Ilies; Nicolae (Bucharest, RO)

  Assignee(s): Cooperativa Agricola DE Productie Scornicesti (judetul Olt, Ro)

  Patent Number: 4,405,602

  Date filed: September 21, 1981

  Abstract: A new process is disclosed for the preparation of a biologically active bee product under sterile conditions. In the process drone bee larvae, worker bee larvae or queen bee larvae are picked up before respective cell capping together with larval food contained in comb cells to form a mixture of crude larval triturate. The mixture is then triturated and filtered to remove impurities to yield the desired product. The product is useful as an animal feed and in the preparation of **royal jelly.**

  Excerpt(s): The present invention relates to a process for the preparation of a biologically active bee-product meant as food, containing vitalizing and regenerating substances, mainly amino-acids, hormones, vitamins and mineral salts. Use can also be made of the said process as described by the invention in order to obtain a bee-product employed as a most biologically active raw material in the apitherapeutic and cosmetic industry. It is known that the food the nurse bees give to the three categories of individuals: queen bee, worker bee and drone, during the first days of their embryonic development, is of identical quality and is known as **royal jelly** which is a purely glandular secretion greatly influencing their entire later metamorphosis in the larval and pupal stages. After a first three-day long post-embryonic stage the worker and drone larvae are offered a kind of food which is qualitativety different from the **royal jelly,** consisting of a nutritive mixture made of pollen, bee bread, honey and water (the worker develops from a fertilized egg and the drone from a non-fertilized one).

  Web site: http://www.delphion.com/details?pn=US04405602__

- **Royal jelly**

  Inventor(s): Bengsch; Eberhard (Olivet, FR)

  Assignee(s): Gsf-forschungszentrum Fur Umwelt Und Gesundheit Gmbh (oberschleissheim, De)

  Patent Number: 5,580,297

  Date filed: March 1, 1995

  Abstract: In a method of extracting **royal jelly** from comb cells of queens, workers, and drones of Apis mellifera, the **royal jelly** is extracted under an inert gas cover such that it does not come into contact with air in the process, whereby the properties of the **royal jelly** are consistently retained.

  Excerpt(s): This is a Continuation-in-Part application of International Application PCT/EP93/02562 filed Sep. 22, 1993 claiming the priority of German application P 42 32 732.6 of Sep. 30, 1992. The invention resides in a standardized **Royal Jelly,** a method of its extraction and the use thereof. It is known that the workers of Apis mellifera generate, between their 9.sup.th and 15.sup.th days of life, a milk-like protein-rich feed juice (royal jelly) in their hypopharyngal glands and especially in the middle mandibular gland. This feed juice is used in small amounts for the original feeding of the whole breed in the egg-containing cells, (worker and drone cells). It is supplied in substantial amounts to the cell in which a queen is to develop whose only purpose is to reproduce. **Royal jelly** is the only food fed to the queen and is completely metabolized by her without excretion. It protects the queen from infection and gives her a life span of 50 times that of normal bees (inspite of the fact that her genes are identical to those of the worker bees). It also endows her with enormous reproductive capacity; up to two million offspring from the initial fertilization.

Web site: http://www.delphion.com/details?pn=US05580297__

- **Scalp treatment composition**

Inventor(s): Hua; Wang Y. (Cheng Du, CN)

Assignee(s): Park; Jerry Y. (houston, Tx)

Patent Number: 5,108,749

Date filed: December 21, 1989

Abstract: A scalp treatment composition which promotes scalp and hair health and growth was developed in China and approved by medical authorities of the Peoples republic of China. The composition consists essentially of ginger (zingiber officianale), saffron (crocus sativus), root bark of shaggy-fruited dittany (orignum dictamnus), the roots of red-rooted salvia (clary or sage), cypress (cypressus semptervirens) leaves, xiang tong (cinnamornum camphora (linn) sieb.), Chinese angelica (aralia chinesis), Sichuan chili (cheilitis), bezoar (phytobezoar), artemisia argyi or Chinese mugworth, **royal jelly** (exudated queen bee), the dried rhizome of rehmannia (scrophulariacae), bear's gallbladder, lard (saturated animal fat), dragon's (daemonorops droco bl.), dragon's blood, gypsum (calcium sulfate), loess (yellowish greay Loam), radix (etymon root), salt (sodium chloride), tuber of multiflower knotweed (centaurer), Chuan poshi (cudrania cochinohinensis (lour) kudo et masam), blended together in a skin permeating agent, e.g., cudrania trienspidata (carr) bur. Through survey and clinical observation, it was found that the effectiveness of this composition to various alopecia reaches 96.82% and to hair loss caused by adipose ooze, 89.82%. The composition is non-poisonous, non harmful and has no side-effect. This composition was the first to pass the inspection of the Chinese Cosmetic Inspection Law since its enactment.

Excerpt(s): This application claims priority from patent application No. 88 1 08860 9 of the Peoples Republic of China. This invention relates generally to a scalp treatment composition which promotes scalp and hair health and growth. The prior art includes many patents disclosing hair grooming compositions which illustrate the state of the art in herbal based compositions for promoting scalp and hair health and growth.

Web site: http://www.delphion.com/details?pn=US05108749__

Patent Applications on Royal Jelly

As of December 2000, U.S. patent applications are open to public viewing.[6] Applications are patent requests which have yet to be granted. (The process to achieve a patent can take several years.) The following patent applications have been filed since December 2000 relating to royal jelly:

---

[6] This has been a common practice outside the United States prior to December 2000.

- **Cell activator**

Inventor(s): Miyake, Toshio; (Okayama, JP)

Correspondence: Browdy & Neimark; Suite 300; 624 Ninth Street NW; Washington; DC; 20001-5303; US

Patent Application Number: 20030059479

Date filed: August 15, 2002

Abstract: The object of the present invention is to provide a daily usable manes for exerting the tonic action inherent to royal jellies, and is solved by providing a cell activating agent comprising a **royal jelly** and trehalose.

Excerpt(s): The present invention relates to a novel cell activating agent, more particularly, to a cell activating agent comprising a **royal jelly** and trehalose. Royal jelly is a white milky secretion from exocrine glands of worker bees, which is accumulated in the royal cell in bees' nests and fed to a larva to be grown up into a queen bee. The larva, that is undistinguishable from other worker bees when it ecloses in the royal cell, grows into a queen bee that has a larger size and a longer life-span than those of worker bees, as well as having a high egg-productivity after having been grown up on a sufficient amount of **royal jelly**. Based on this, **royal jelly** has been recognized to have a variety of physiological functions such as tonicity and promotion of stamina. For example, it is described in Shikou Bessatsu-Honey-Book (titled "Preference" in special edition of "Meidi-ya's Honey Book"), page 22, published by Meidi-Ya Honsha, 1965, that "Royal jelly may have distinctive medical effects such that it augments physical strength and stamina, improves skin activity, and turns gray hairs into black". Since **royal jelly** is a natural product, it would be substantially free from serious side effect if taken by mammals including humans. Based on these, the application of **royal jelly** for exerting tonicity has been greatly expected that it would overcome unfavorable side effect frequently found in conventional tonics. However, **royal jelly** has the drawback that it easily deteriorates when in an intact form just after collection and then promptly loses its inherent actions. To overcome the defect, **royal jelly** is preserved at temperatures lower than 0.degree. C. or at lower temperatures thereabout or used after dryness. These treatments may exert a comparatively effective inhibitory action on quality deterioration of **royal jelly** during storage, but have troublesome in its handling during preservation at lower temperatures. The dryness of **royal jelly** would inevitably deteriorate the inherent quality of **royal jelly** during its processing, and this hinders sufficient exertion of the inherent action of **royal jelly**. As described above, in spite of its expectation, **royal jelly** could not be said to have been being used as a tonic easily and effectively.

Web site: http://appft1.uspto.gov/netahtml/PTO/search-bool.html

- **Drinks consisting of extracts of fomes japonicus extracted with honey and vinegar**

Inventor(s): Ishikawa, Takeshi; (Hiroshima-shi, JP), Sumihara, Kazuhiko; (Hiroshima-Shi, JP)

Correspondence: Oblon, Spivak, Mcclelland, Maier & Neustadt, P.C.; 1940 Duke Street; Alexandria; VA; 22314; US

Patent Application Number: 20030096049

Date filed: September 6, 2002

Abstract: A Fomes japonicus extract is prepared by extracting Fomes japonicus with a mixture of honey and vinegar, heating the resulting extract to a temperature of not less than 95.degree. C. and then filtering the heated extract. The Fomes japonicus extract can be diluted with water to give a drink such as a health beverage. Moreover, the addition of **royal jelly** to the extract permits the preparation of a royal jelly-supplemented drink additionally having nutritive and restorative effects.

Excerpt(s): The present application is a continuation of provisional application Serial No. 60/327,031 filed Oct. 5, 2001. The present invention relates to a method for preparing a Fomes japonicus extract, which emits only a reduced odor of acetic acid and which is free of any turbidity, as well as to a method for preparing a drink obtained from the Fomes japonicus extract. Fomes japonicus (REISHI) is a kind of mushroom also called the bracket fungus of the genus Fomes belonging to the family Polyporaceae. The plant has been used in the past for a variety of therapeutic properties attributed to consumption of the plant including improvement of the blood circulation; the prevention of, for instance, headaches, anemia, oversensitivity to the cold and allergic diseases; relief of fatigue; as well as a carcinostatic effect. Fomes japonicus has been highly prized as a Chinese herbal remedy.

Web site: http://appft1.uspto.gov/netahtml/PTO/search-bool.html

Method of treatment

Inventor(s): Hedman, Christer; (Molnlycke, SE), Karnerud, Lars; (Tenhult, SE), Winter, Kaj; (Copenhagen, DK)

Correspondence: Browdy And Neimark, P.L.L.C.; 624 Ninth Street, NW; Suite 300; Washington; DC; 20001-5303; US

Patent Application Number: 20020061337

Date filed: August 31, 2001

Abstract: A method for the treatment of symptoms related to normal hormonal variations in women during fertile, peri- and post-menopausal age, by the administering of a composition comprising, as active ingredients, a water and/or fat-soluble cytosolic extract of pollen, optionally combined with **Royal Jelly** and Vitamin

Excerpt(s): The invention relates in a first aspect to a method for the treatment of symptoms related to normal hormonal variations in women during fertile as well as, peri- and post-menopausal age, by the administering of a composition comprising, as active ingredients, a water and/or fat soluble cytosolic extract of pollen, optionally combined with **Royal Jelly** and Vitamin E. The invention, in another aspect, relates to the use of a composition comprising, as active ingredients, a water and/or fat soluble extract of pollen optionally combined with **Royal Jelly** and Vitamin E for the manufacturing of a medicament for the treatment of symptoms relating to normal hormonal variations in women during fertile, as well as peri- and post-menopausal age. An extract of combined pollen and pistils combined with a pollen grain extract, **Royal Jelly** and Vitamin B has been sold by Interhealth AB, Kungsngsvgen 27, 561 56 Huskvarna, Sweden, for the treatment of Pre-Menstrual Syndrome (PMS). Said composition was thought to be active against PMS symptoms in general but the present inventors during research work found out that the composition as disclosed in the application showed an unexpected advantageous effect on some symptoms relating to normal variations in the hormone cycle of women. Other symptoms, such as heart rate and blood pressure, remain unaffected of the remedy.

Web site: http://appft1.uspto.gov/netahtml/PTO/search-bool.html

- **Method of treatment**

Inventor(s): Hedman, Christer; (Molnlycke, SE), Karnerud, Lars; (Tenhult, SE), Winter, Kaj; (Copenhage, DK)

Correspondence: Browdy And Neimark, P.L.L.C.; 624 Ninth Street, N.W.; Washington; DC; 20001; US

Patent Application Number: 20030161890

Date filed: June 28, 2002

Abstract: A method for the treatment of disorders related to normal hormonal variations in women during fertile, peri- and post-menopausal age, by the administering of a composition comprising, as active ingredients, a water and/or fat-soluble cytosolic extract of pollen and optionally pistils, optionally combined with **Royal Jelly** and vitamin E.

Excerpt(s): The invention relates in a first aspect to a method for the treatment of disorders related to normal hormonal variations in women during fertile as well as, peri- and post-menopausal age, by the administering of a composition comprising, as active ingredients, a water- and/or fat-soluble cytosolic extract of pollen and optionally pistils. The invention, in another aspect, relates to a composition comprising, as active ingredients, a water- and/or fat-soluble cytosolic extract of pollen and optionally pistils for the treatment of disorders relating to normal hormonal variations in women during fertile, as well as peri- and post-menopausal age. Disorders relating to normal variation of the sex hormone cycle of women of fertile age are tension, irritability, dysphoria, abdominal distension or bloatedness, severe breast tension, headache or migraine, edema, weight changes, sleep disturbances etc. The overall well being as well as the social and professional life may be influenced.

Web site: http://appft1.uspto.gov/netahtml/PTO/search-bool.html

- **Royal jelly collection frame**

Inventor(s): Jang, Bong Hwan; (Seo-gu, KR)

Correspondence: Bacon & Thomas, Pllc; 625 Slaters Lane; Fourth Floor; Alexandria; VA; 22314

Patent Application Number: 20020137429

Date filed: March 15, 2002

Abstract: The invention relates to a **royal jelly** collection frame which enables to cultivate the queen bees easily and to collect **royal jelly** productively. According to the invention, there is provided with a **royal jelly** collection frame (10) comprising of a queen excluder panel (2) having a plurality of holes through which the working bee can pass but the queen bee can not pass and a queen bee passage window (3) into which the queen bee can pass and it could be closed by cover, a queen cup insert panel (4) being spaced from the queen excluder panel (2) and having a plurality of hollow projections (21) into which the queen bee may spawn, an single queen cup member (5) having an closed end and being insertable into the outer wall of the hollow projections (21), and a bundle queen cup member (6) having a plurality of queen cup and being insertable into the corresponding hollow projections (21), and at least a queen cup mount (1) disposed at the other part of frame (10) and into which the bundle queen cup member can be mounted.

Excerpt(s): The present invention relates to a **royal jelly** collection frame, and more particularly to a **royal jelly** collection frame which enables to bring up the queen bees easily and to collect **royal jelly** productively. The success of bee keeping mainly depends upon how to acquire many superior queen bees, so the bee-keeper makes efforts to cultivate superior queen bee. In order to cultivate queen bees, the larvae of bee should be moved from the small working bee cells of honeycomb to the relatively big artificial queen cups in which the larvae will grow into queen bees or the working bee will secrete **royal jelly.** To do this, the bee keeper should cautiously pick up the individual larva by needle or pincette manually to move it without causing no damage on larva. And it will be impossible for the weak-sighted bee keeper to move the larvae from working bee cells to queen cups without causing the wounds on larvae. Therefore, the job of moving the larvae is very difficult and troublesome, so requires many times and labors. On the other hand, in order to collect the **royal jelly,** it is also necessary to transfer many larvae from working bee cells into queen cups, which will also cause many labors and times. Therefore, it is desired to provide a solution to move the larvae from working bee cells to queen cups effectively for cultivating the queen bee or for collecting **royal jelly.**

Web site: http://appft1.uspto.gov/netahtml/PTO/search-bool.html

Keeping Current

In order to stay informed about patents and patent applications dealing with royal jelly, you can access the U.S. Patent Office archive via the Internet at the following Web address: **http://www.uspto.gov/patft/index.html**. You will see two broad options: (1) Issued Patent, and (2) Published Applications. To see a list of issued patents, perform the following steps: Under "Issued Patents," click "Quick Search." Then, type "royal jelly" (or synonyms) into the "Term 1" box. After clicking on the search button, scroll down to see the various patents which have been granted to date on royal jelly.

You can also use this procedure to view pending patent applications concerning royal jelly. Simply go back to **http://www.uspto.gov/patft/index.html**. Select "Quick Search" under "Published Applications." Then proceed with the steps listed above.

CHAPTER 5. BOOKS ON ROYAL JELLY

Overview

This chapter provides bibliographic book references relating to royal jelly. In addition to online booksellers such as **www.amazon.com** and **www.bn.com**, excellent sources for book titles on royal jelly include the Combined Health Information Database and the National Library of Medicine. Your local medical library also may have these titles available for loan.

Book Summaries: Online Booksellers

Commercial Internet-based booksellers, such as Amazon.com and Barnes&Noble.com, offer summaries which have been supplied by each title's publisher. Some summaries also include customer reviews. Your local bookseller may have access to in-house and commercial databases that index all published books (e.g. Books in Print®). **IMPORTANT NOTE:** Online booksellers typically produce search results for medical and non-medical books. When searching for "royal jelly" at online booksellers' Web sites, you may discover <u>non-medical books</u> that use the generic term "royal jelly" (or a synonym) in their titles. The following is indicative of the results you might find when searching for "royal jelly" (sorted alphabetically by title; follow the hyperlink to view more details at Amazon.com):

- **Bee Pollen, Royal Jelly, Propolis and Honey: An Extraordinary Energy and Health-Promoting Ensemble (Woodland Health Series)** by Rita Elkins; ISBN: 1885670125; http://www.amazon.com/exec/obidos/ASIN/1885670125/icongroupinterna

- **Bee Well - Bee Wise : with bee pollen, propolis, and royal jelly** by Bernard Jensen; ISBN: 0932615309; http://www.amazon.com/exec/obidos/ASIN/0932615309/icongroupinterna

- **Health from the Hive: Honey.Bee Pollen.Bee Propolis.Royal Jelly** by Carlson Wade; ISBN: 0879835818; http://www.amazon.com/exec/obidos/ASIN/0879835818/icongroupinterna

- **Royal Jelly**; ISBN: 0722512252; http://www.amazon.com/exec/obidos/ASIN/0722512252/icongroupinterna

- **ROYAL JELLY - SPECIAL EDITION**; ISBN: 0722521723; http://www.amazon.com/exec/obidos/ASIN/0722521723/icongroupinterna

- **ROYAL JELLY (EBURY SPEC SALES)**; ISBN: 0091861772;
  http://www.amazon.com/exec/obidos/ASIN/0091861772/icongroupinterna

- **Royal Jelly: The New Guide to Nature's Richest Health Food** by Irene Stein; ISBN: 0722521596;
  http://www.amazon.com/exec/obidos/ASIN/0722521596/icongroupinterna

- **The Healing Power of Pollen With Propolis and Royal Jelly** by Maurice Hanssen; ISBN: 0722505264;
  http://www.amazon.com/exec/obidos/ASIN/0722505264/icongroupinterna

- **The Longevity Solution: Compelling Proof That Royal Jelly Has the Power to Eliminate Fatigue, Provide Greater Energy and Extend Life** by Cass, Dr Ingram; ISBN: 1931078017;
  http://www.amazon.com/exec/obidos/ASIN/1931078017/icongroupinterna

- **The Royal Jelly Miracle** by Reynalud, Dr. Allen, et al; ISBN: 0879040238;
  http://www.amazon.com/exec/obidos/ASIN/0879040238/icongroupinterna

- **Three Ways to Total Health: Ginseng, Evening Primrose Oil, Royal Jelly** by Vernon Lloyd-Jones LCSP; ISBN: 0715407260;
  http://www.amazon.com/exec/obidos/ASIN/0715407260/icongroupinterna

Chapters on Royal Jelly

In order to find chapters that specifically relate to royal jelly, an excellent source of abstracts is the Combined Health Information Database. You will need to limit your search to book chapters and royal jelly using the "Detailed Search" option. Go to the following hyperlink: **http://chid.nih.gov/detail/detail.html**. To find book chapters, use the drop boxes at the bottom of the search page where "You may refine your search by." Select the dates and language you prefer, and the format option "Book Chapter." Type "royal jelly" (or synonyms) into the "For these words:" box.

APPENDICES

APPENDIX A. PHYSICIAN RESOURCES

Overview

In this chapter, we focus on databases and Internet-based guidelines and information resources created or written for a professional audience.

NIH Guidelines

Commonly referred to as "clinical" or "professional" guidelines, the National Institutes of Health publish physician guidelines for the most common diseases. Publications are available at the following by relevant Institute[7]:

- Office of the Director (OD); guidelines consolidated across agencies available at **http://www.nih.gov/health/consumer/conkey.htm**

- National Institute of General Medical Sciences (NIGMS); fact sheets available at **http://www.nigms.nih.gov/news/facts/**

- National Library of Medicine (NLM); extensive encyclopedia (A.D.A.M., Inc.) with guidelines: **http://www.nlm.nih.gov/medlineplus/healthtopics.html**

- National Cancer Institute (NCI); guidelines available at **http://www.cancer.gov/cancerinfo/list.aspx?viewid=5f35036e-5497-4d86-8c2c-714a9f7c8d25**

- National Eye Institute (NEI); guidelines available at **http://www.nei.nih.gov/order/index.htm**

- National Heart, Lung, and Blood Institute (NHLBI); guidelines available at **http://www.nhlbi.nih.gov/guidelines/index.htm**

- National Human Genome Research Institute (NHGRI); research available at **http://www.genome.gov/page.cfm?pageID=10000375**

- National Institute on Aging (NIA); guidelines available at **http://www.nia.nih.gov/health/**

---

[7] These publications are typically written by one or more of the various NIH Institutes.

- National Institute on Alcohol Abuse and Alcoholism (NIAAA); guidelines available at http://www.niaaa.nih.gov/publications/publications.htm

- National Institute of Allergy and Infectious Diseases (NIAID); guidelines available at http://www.niaid.nih.gov/publications/

- National Institute of Arthritis and Musculoskeletal and Skin Diseases (NIAMS); fact sheets and guidelines available at http://www.niams.nih.gov/hi/index.htm

- National Institute of Child Health and Human Development (NICHD); guidelines available at http://www.nichd.nih.gov/publications/pubskey.cfm

- National Institute on Deafness and Other Communication Disorders (NIDCD); fact sheets and guidelines at http://www.nidcd.nih.gov/health/

- National Institute of Dental and Craniofacial Research (NIDCR); guidelines available at http://www.nidr.nih.gov/health/

- National Institute of Diabetes and Digestive and Kidney Diseases (NIDDK); guidelines available at http://www.niddk.nih.gov/health/health.htm

- National Institute on Drug Abuse (NIDA); guidelines available at http://www.nida.nih.gov/DrugAbuse.html

- National Institute of Environmental Health Sciences (NIEHS); environmental health information available at http://www.niehs.nih.gov/external/facts.htm

- National Institute of Mental Health (NIMH); guidelines available at http://www.nimh.nih.gov/practitioners/index.cfm

- National Institute of Neurological Disorders and Stroke (NINDS); neurological disorder information pages available at http://www.ninds.nih.gov/health_and_medical/disorder_index.htm

- National Institute of Nursing Research (NINR); publications on selected illnesses at http://www.nih.gov/ninr/news-info/publications.html

- National Institute of Biomedical Imaging and Bioengineering; general information at http://grants.nih.gov/grants/becon/becon_info.htm

- Center for Information Technology (CIT); referrals to other agencies based on keyword searches available at http://kb.nih.gov/www_query_main.asp

- National Center for Complementary and Alternative Medicine (NCCAM); health information available at http://nccam.nih.gov/health/

- National Center for Research Resources (NCRR); various information directories available at http://www.ncrr.nih.gov/publications.asp

- Office of Rare Diseases; various fact sheets available at http://rarediseases.info.nih.gov/html/resources/rep_pubs.html

- Centers for Disease Control and Prevention; various fact sheets on infectious diseases available at http://www.cdc.gov/publications.htm

NIH Databases

In addition to the various Institutes of Health that publish professional guidelines, the NIH has designed a number of databases for professionals.[8] Physician-oriented resources provide a wide variety of information related to the biomedical and health sciences, both past and present. The format of these resources varies. Searchable databases, bibliographic citations, full-text articles (when available), archival collections, and images are all available. The following are referenced by the National Library of Medicine:[9]

- **Bioethics:** Access to published literature on the ethical, legal, and public policy issues surrounding healthcare and biomedical research. This information is provided in conjunction with the Kennedy Institute of Ethics located at Georgetown University, Washington, D.C.: **http://www.nlm.nih.gov/databases/databases_bioethics.html**

- **HIV/AIDS Resources:** Describes various links and databases dedicated to HIV/AIDS research: **http://www.nlm.nih.gov/pubs/factsheets/aidsinfs.html**

- **NLM Online Exhibitions:** Describes "Exhibitions in the History of Medicine": **http://www.nlm.nih.gov/exhibition/exhibition.html**. Additional resources for historical scholarship in medicine: **http://www.nlm.nih.gov/hmd/hmd.html**

- **Biotechnology Information:** Access to public databases. The National Center for Biotechnology Information conducts research in computational biology, develops software tools for analyzing genome data, and disseminates biomedical information for the better understanding of molecular processes affecting human health and disease: **http://www.ncbi.nlm.nih.gov/**

- **Population Information:** The National Library of Medicine provides access to worldwide coverage of population, family planning, and related health issues, including family planning technology and programs, fertility, and population law and policy: **http://www.nlm.nih.gov/databases/databases_population.html**

- **Cancer Information:** Access to cancer-oriented databases: **http://www.nlm.nih.gov/databases/databases_cancer.html**

- **Profiles in Science:** Offering the archival collections of prominent twentieth-century biomedical scientists to the public through modern digital technology: **http://www.profiles.nlm.nih.gov/**

- **Chemical Information:** Provides links to various chemical databases and references: **http://sis.nlm.nih.gov/Chem/ChemMain.html**

- **Clinical Alerts:** Reports the release of findings from the NIH-funded clinical trials where such release could significantly affect morbidity and mortality: **http://www.nlm.nih.gov/databases/alerts/clinical_alerts.html**

- **Space Life Sciences:** Provides links and information to space-based research (including NASA): **http://www.nlm.nih.gov/databases/databases_space.html**

- **MEDLINE:** Bibliographic database covering the fields of medicine, nursing, dentistry, veterinary medicine, the healthcare system, and the pre-clinical sciences: **http://www.nlm.nih.gov/databases/databases_medline.html**

---

[8] Remember, for the general public, the National Library of Medicine recommends the databases referenced in MEDLINE*plus* (**http://medlineplus.gov/** or **http://www.nlm.nih.gov/medlineplus/databases.html**).

[9] See **http://www.nlm.nih.gov/databases/databases.html**.

- **Toxicology and Environmental Health Information (TOXNET):** Databases covering toxicology and environmental health: **http://sis.nlm.nih.gov/Tox/ToxMain.html**

- **Visible Human Interface:** Anatomically detailed, three-dimensional representations of normal male and female human bodies: **http://www.nlm.nih.gov/research/visible/visible_human.html**

The NLM Gateway[10]

The NLM (National Library of Medicine) Gateway is a Web-based system that lets users search simultaneously in multiple retrieval systems at the U.S. National Library of Medicine (NLM). It allows users of NLM services to initiate searches from one Web interface, providing one-stop searching for many of NLM's information resources or databases.[11] To use the NLM Gateway, simply go to the search site at **http://gateway.nlm.nih.gov/gw/Cmd**. Type "royal jelly" (or synonyms) into the search box and click "Search." The results will be presented in a tabular form, indicating the number of references in each database category.

Results Summary

Category	Items Found
Journal Articles	297
Books / Periodicals / Audio Visual	See Details
Consumer Health	93
Meeting Abstracts	0
Other Collections	0
Total	390

HSTAT[12]

HSTAT is a free, Web-based resource that provides access to full-text documents used in healthcare decision-making.[13] These documents include clinical practice guidelines, quick-reference guides for clinicians, consumer health brochures, evidence reports and technology assessments from the Agency for Healthcare Research and Quality (AHRQ), as well as AHRQ's Put Prevention Into Practice.[14] Simply search by "royal jelly" (or synonyms) at the following Web site: **http://text.nlm.nih.gov.**

---

[10] Adapted from NLM: **http://gateway.nlm.nih.gov/gw/Cmd?Overview.x.**

[11] The NLM Gateway is currently being developed by the Lister Hill National Center for Biomedical Communications (LHNCBC) at the National Library of Medicine (NLM) of the National Institutes of Health (NIH).

[12] Adapted from HSTAT: **http://www.nlm.nih.gov/pubs/factsheets/hstat.html.**

[13] The HSTAT URL is **http://hstat.nlm.nih.gov/.**

[14] Other important documents in HSTAT include: the National Institutes of Health (NIH) Consensus Conference Reports and Technology Assessment Reports; the HIV/AIDS Treatment Information Service (ATIS) resource documents; the Substance Abuse and Mental Health Services Administration's Center for Substance Abuse Treatment (SAMHSA/CSAT) Treatment Improvement Protocols (TIP) and Center for Substance Abuse Prevention (SAMHSA/CSAP) Prevention Enhancement Protocols System (PEPS); the Public Health Service (PHS) Preventive Services Task Force's *Guide to Clinical Preventive Services*; the independent, nonfederal Task Force on Community Services' *Guide to Community Preventive Services*; and the Health Technology Advisory Committee (HTAC) of the Minnesota Health Care Commission (MHCC) health technology evaluations.

Coffee Break: Tutorials for Biologists[15]

Coffee Break is a general healthcare site that takes a scientific view of the news and covers recent breakthroughs in biology that may one day assist physicians in developing treatments. Here you will find a collection of short reports on recent biological discoveries. Each report incorporates interactive tutorials that demonstrate how bioinformatics tools are used as a part of the research process. Currently, all Coffee Breaks are written by NCBI staff.[16] Each report is about 400 words and is usually based on a discovery reported in one or more articles from recently published, peer-reviewed literature.[17] This site has new articles every few weeks, so it can be considered an online magazine of sorts. It is intended for general background information. You can access the Coffee Break Web site at the following hyperlink: **http://www.ncbi.nlm.nih.gov/Coffeebreak/**.

Other Commercial Databases

In addition to resources maintained by official agencies, other databases exist that are commercial ventures addressing medical professionals. Here are some examples that may interest you:

- **CliniWeb International:** Index and table of contents to selected clinical information on the Internet; see **http://www.ohsu.edu/cliniweb/**.

- **Medical World Search:** Searches full text from thousands of selected medical sites on the Internet; see **http://www.mwsearch.com/**.

---

[15] Adapted from **http://www.ncbi.nlm.nih.gov/Coffeebreak/Archive/FAQ.html**.

[16] The figure that accompanies each article is frequently supplied by an expert external to NCBI, in which case the source of the figure is cited. The result is an interactive tutorial that tells a biological story.

[17] After a brief introduction that sets the work described into a broader context, the report focuses on how a molecular understanding can provide explanations of observed biology and lead to therapies for diseases. Each vignette is accompanied by a figure and hypertext links that lead to a series of pages that interactively show how NCBI tools and resources are used in the research process.

APPENDIX B. PATIENT RESOURCES

Overview

Official agencies, as well as federally funded institutions supported by national grants, frequently publish a variety of guidelines written with the patient in mind. These are typically called "Fact Sheets" or "Guidelines." They can take the form of a brochure, information kit, pamphlet, or flyer. Often they are only a few pages in length. Since new guidelines on royal jelly can appear at any moment and be published by a number of sources, the best approach to finding guidelines is to systematically scan the Internet-based services that post them.

Patient Guideline Sources

The remainder of this chapter directs you to sources which either publish or can help you find additional guidelines on topics related to royal jelly. Due to space limitations, these sources are listed in a concise manner. Do not hesitate to consult the following sources by either using the Internet hyperlink provided, or, in cases where the contact information is provided, contacting the publisher or author directly.

The National Institutes of Health

The NIH gateway to patients is located at **http://health.nih.gov/**. From this site, you can search across various sources and institutes, a number of which are summarized below.

Topic Pages: MEDLINEplus

The National Library of Medicine has created a vast and patient-oriented healthcare information portal called MEDLINEplus. Within this Internet-based system are "health topic pages" which list links to available materials relevant to royal jelly. To access this system, log on to **http://www.nlm.nih.gov/medlineplus/healthtopics.html**. From there you can either search using the alphabetical index or browse by broad topic areas. Recently, MEDLINEplus listed the following when searched for "royal jelly":

- Other guides

  Dietary Supplements
  http://www.nlm.nih.gov/medlineplus/dietarysupplements.html

  Food Safety
  http://www.nlm.nih.gov/medlineplus/foodsafety.html

  Plastic and Cosmetic Surgery
  http://www.nlm.nih.gov/medlineplus/plasticandcosmeticsurgery.html

  Vitamins and Minerals
  http://www.nlm.nih.gov/medlineplus/vitaminsandminerals.html

You may also choose to use the search utility provided by MEDLINEplus at the following Web address: **http://www.nlm.nih.gov/medlineplus/**. Simply type a keyword into the search box and click "Search." This utility is similar to the NIH search utility, with the exception that it only includes materials that are linked within the MEDLINEplus system (mostly patient-oriented information). It also has the disadvantage of generating unstructured results. We recommend, therefore, that you use this method only if you have a very targeted search.

The NIH Search Utility

The NIH search utility allows you to search for documents on over 100 selected Web sites that comprise the NIH-WEB-SPACE. Each of these servers is "crawled" and indexed on an ongoing basis. Your search will produce a list of various documents, all of which will relate in some way to royal jelly. The drawbacks of this approach are that the information is not organized by theme and that the references are often a mix of information for professionals and patients. Nevertheless, a large number of the listed Web sites provide useful background information. We can only recommend this route, therefore, for relatively rare or specific disorders, or when using highly targeted searches. To use the NIH search utility, visit the following Web page: **http://search.nih.gov/index.html**.

Additional Web Sources

A number of Web sites are available to the public that often link to government sites. These can also point you in the direction of essential information. The following is a representative sample:

- AOL: **http://search.aol.com/cat.adp?id=168&layer=&from=subcats**

- Family Village: **http://www.familyvillage.wisc.edu/specific.htm**

- Google: **http://directory.google.com/Top/Health/Conditions_and_Diseases/**

- Med Help International: **http://www.medhelp.org/HealthTopics/A.html**

- Open Directory Project: **http://dmoz.org/Health/Conditions_and_Diseases/**

- Yahoo.com: **http://dir.yahoo.com/Health/Diseases_and_Conditions/**

- WebMD®Health: **http://my.webmd.com/health_topics**

Finding Associations

There are several Internet directories that provide lists of medical associations with information on or resources relating to royal jelly. By consulting all of associations listed in this chapter, you will have nearly exhausted all sources for patient associations concerned with royal jelly.

The National Health Information Center (NHIC)

The National Health Information Center (NHIC) offers a free referral service to help people find organizations that provide information about royal jelly. For more information, see the NHIC's Web site at **http://www.health.gov/NHIC/** or contact an information specialist by calling 1-800-336-4797.

Directory of Health Organizations

The Directory of Health Organizations, provided by the National Library of Medicine Specialized Information Services, is a comprehensive source of information on associations. The Directory of Health Organizations database can be accessed via the Internet at **http://www.sis.nlm.nih.gov/Dir/DirMain.html**. It is composed of two parts: DIRLINE and Health Hotlines.

The DIRLINE database comprises some 10,000 records of organizations, research centers, and government institutes and associations that primarily focus on health and biomedicine. To access DIRLINE directly, go to the following Web site: **http://dirline.nlm.nih.gov/**. Simply type in "royal jelly" (or a synonym), and you will receive information on all relevant organizations listed in the database.

Health Hotlines directs you to toll-free numbers to over 300 organizations. You can access this database directly at **http://www.sis.nlm.nih.gov/hotlines/**. On this page, you are given the option to search by keyword or by browsing the subject list. When you have received your search results, click on the name of the organization for its description and contact information.

The Combined Health Information Database

Another comprehensive source of information on healthcare associations is the Combined Health Information Database. Using the "Detailed Search" option, you will need to limit your search to "Organizations" and "royal jelly". Type the following hyperlink into your Web browser: **http://chid.nih.gov/detail/detail.html**. To find associations, use the drop boxes at the bottom of the search page where "You may refine your search by." For publication date, select "All Years." Then, select your preferred language and the format option "Organization Resource Sheet." Type "royal jelly" (or synonyms) into the "For these words:" box. You should check back periodically with this database since it is updated every three months.

The National Organization for Rare Disorders, Inc.

The National Organization for Rare Disorders, Inc. has prepared a Web site that provides, at no charge, lists of associations organized by health topic. You can access this database at the following Web site: **http://www.rarediseases.org/search/orgsearch.html**. Type "royal jelly" (or a synonym) into the search box, and click "Submit Query."

APPENDIX C. FINDING MEDICAL LIBRARIES

Overview

In this Appendix, we show you how to quickly find a medical library in your area.

Preparation

Your local public library and medical libraries have interlibrary loan programs with the National Library of Medicine (NLM), one of the largest medical collections in the world. According to the NLM, most of the literature in the general and historical collections of the National Library of Medicine is available on interlibrary loan to any library. If you would like to access NLM medical literature, then visit a library in your area that can request the publications for you.[18]

Finding a Local Medical Library

The quickest method to locate medical libraries is to use the Internet-based directory published by the National Network of Libraries of Medicine (NN/LM). This network includes 4626 members and affiliates that provide many services to librarians, health professionals, and the public. To find a library in your area, simply visit **http://nnlm.gov/members/adv.html** or call 1-800-338-7657.

Medical Libraries in the U.S. and Canada

In addition to the NN/LM, the National Library of Medicine (NLM) lists a number of libraries with reference facilities that are open to the public. The following is the NLM's list and includes hyperlinks to each library's Web site. These Web pages can provide information on hours of operation and other restrictions. The list below is a small sample of

---

[18] Adapted from the NLM: **http://www.nlm.nih.gov/psd/cas/interlibrary.html**.

libraries recommended by the National Library of Medicine (sorted alphabetically by name of the U.S. state or Canadian province where the library is located)[19]:

- **Alabama:** Health InfoNet of Jefferson County (Jefferson County Library Cooperative, Lister Hill Library of the Health Sciences), **http://www.uab.edu/infonet/**

- **Alabama:** Richard M. Scrushy Library (American Sports Medicine Institute)

- **Arizona:** Samaritan Regional Medical Center: The Learning Center (Samaritan Health System, Phoenix, Arizona), **http://www.samaritan.edu/library/bannerlibs.htm**

- **California:** Kris Kelly Health Information Center (St. Joseph Health System, Humboldt), **http://www.humboldt1.com/~kkhic/index.html**

- **California:** Community Health Library of Los Gatos, **http://www.healthlib.org/orgresources.html**

- **California:** Consumer Health Program and Services (CHIPS) (County of Los Angeles Public Library, Los Angeles County Harbor-UCLA Medical Center Library) - Carson, CA, **http://www.colapublib.org/services/chips.html**

- **California:** Gateway Health Library (Sutter Gould Medical Foundation)

- **California:** Health Library (Stanford University Medical Center), **http://www-med.stanford.edu/healthlibrary/**

- **California:** Patient Education Resource Center - Health Information and Resources (University of California, San Francisco), **http://sfghdean.ucsf.edu/barnett/PERC/default.asp**

- **California:** Redwood Health Library (Petaluma Health Care District), **http://www.phcd.org/rdwdlib.html**

- **California:** Los Gatos PlaneTree Health Library, **http://planetreesanjose.org/**

- **California:** Sutter Resource Library (Sutter Hospitals Foundation, Sacramento), **http://suttermedicalcenter.org/library/**

- **California:** Health Sciences Libraries (University of California, Davis), **http://www.lib.ucdavis.edu/healthsci/**

- **California:** ValleyCare Health Library & Ryan Comer Cancer Resource Center (ValleyCare Health System, Pleasanton), **http://gaelnet.stmarys-ca.edu/other.libs/gbal/east/vchl.html**

- **California:** Washington Community Health Resource Library (Fremont), **http://www.healthlibrary.org/**

- **Colorado:** William V. Gervasini Memorial Library (Exempla Healthcare), **http://www.saintjosephdenver.org/yourhealth/libraries/**

- **Connecticut:** Hartford Hospital Health Science Libraries (Hartford Hospital), **http://www.harthosp.org/library/**

- **Connecticut:** Healthnet: Connecticut Consumer Health Information Center (University of Connecticut Health Center, Lyman Maynard Stowe Library), **http://library.uchc.edu/departm/hnet/**

[19] Abstracted from **http://www.nlm.nih.gov/medlineplus/libraries.html**.

- **Connecticut:** Waterbury Hospital Health Center Library (Waterbury Hospital, Waterbury), **http://www.waterburyhospital.com/library/consumer.shtml**

- **Delaware:** Consumer Health Library (Christiana Care Health System, Eugene du Pont Preventive Medicine & Rehabilitation Institute, Wilmington), **http://www.christianacare.org/health_guide/health_guide_pmri_health_info.cfm**

- **Delaware:** Lewis B. Flinn Library (Delaware Academy of Medicine, Wilmington), **http://www.delamed.org/chls.html**

- **Georgia:** Family Resource Library (Medical College of Georgia, Augusta), **http://cmc.mcg.edu/kids_families/fam_resources/fam_res_lib/frl.htm**

- **Georgia:** Health Resource Center (Medical Center of Central Georgia, Macon), **http://www.mccg.org/hrc/hrchome.asp**

- **Hawaii:** Hawaii Medical Library: Consumer Health Information Service (Hawaii Medical Library, Honolulu), **http://hml.org/CHIS/**

- **Idaho:** DeArmond Consumer Health Library (Kootenai Medical Center, Coeur d'Alene), **http://www.nicon.org/DeArmond/index.htm**

- **Illinois:** Health Learning Center of Northwestern Memorial Hospital (Chicago), **http://www.nmh.org/health_info/hlc.html**

- **Illinois:** Medical Library (OSF Saint Francis Medical Center, Peoria), **http://www.osfsaintfrancis.org/general/library/**

- **Kentucky:** Medical Library - Services for Patients, Families, Students & the Public (Central Baptist Hospital, Lexington), **http://www.centralbap.com/education/community/library.cfm**

- **Kentucky:** University of Kentucky - Health Information Library (Chandler Medical Center, Lexington), **http://www.mc.uky.edu/PatientEd/**

- **Louisiana:** Alton Ochsner Medical Foundation Library (Alton Ochsner Medical Foundation, New Orleans), **http://www.ochsner.org/library/**

- **Louisiana:** Louisiana State University Health Sciences Center Medical Library-Shreveport, **http://lib-sh.lsuhsc.edu/**

- **Maine:** Franklin Memorial Hospital Medical Library (Franklin Memorial Hospital, Farmington), **http://www.fchn.org/fmh/lib.htm**

- **Maine:** Gerrish-True Health Sciences Library (Central Maine Medical Center, Lewiston), **http://www.cmmc.org/library/library.html**

- **Maine:** Hadley Parrot Health Science Library (Eastern Maine Healthcare, Bangor), **http://www.emh.org/hll/hpl/guide.htm**

- **Maine:** Maine Medical Center Library (Maine Medical Center, Portland), **http://www.mmc.org/library/**

- **Maine:** Parkview Hospital (Brunswick), **http://www.parkviewhospital.org/**

- **Maine:** Southern Maine Medical Center Health Sciences Library (Southern Maine Medical Center, Biddeford), **http://www.smmc.org/services/service.php3?choice=10**

- **Maine:** Stephens Memorial Hospital's Health Information Library (Western Maine Health, Norway), **http://www.wmhcc.org/Library/**

- **Manitoba, Canada:** Consumer & Patient Health Information Service (University of Manitoba Libraries), http://www.umanitoba.ca/libraries/units/health/reference/chis.html

- **Manitoba, Canada:** J.W. Crane Memorial Library (Deer Lodge Centre, Winnipeg), http://www.deerlodge.mb.ca/crane_library/about.asp

- **Maryland:** Health Information Center at the Wheaton Regional Library (Montgomery County, Dept. of Public Libraries, Wheaton Regional Library), http://www.mont.lib.md.us/healthinfo/hic.asp

- **Massachusetts:** Baystate Medical Center Library (Baystate Health System), http://www.baystatehealth.com/1024/

- **Massachusetts:** Boston University Medical Center Alumni Medical Library (Boston University Medical Center), http://med-libwww.bu.edu/library/lib.html

- **Massachusetts:** Lowell General Hospital Health Sciences Library (Lowell General Hospital, Lowell), http://www.lowellgeneral.org/library/HomePageLinks/WWW.htm

- **Massachusetts:** Paul E. Woodard Health Sciences Library (New England Baptist Hospital, Boston), http://www.nebh.org/health_lib.asp

- **Massachusetts:** St. Luke's Hospital Health Sciences Library (St. Luke's Hospital, Southcoast Health System, New Bedford), http://www.southcoast.org/library/

- **Massachusetts:** Treadwell Library Consumer Health Reference Center (Massachusetts General Hospital), http://www.mgh.harvard.edu/library/chrcindex.html

- **Massachusetts:** UMass HealthNet (University of Massachusetts Medical School, Worchester), http://healthnet.umassmed.edu/

- **Michigan:** Botsford General Hospital Library - Consumer Health (Botsford General Hospital, Library & Internet Services), http://www.botsfordlibrary.org/consumer.htm

- **Michigan:** Helen DeRoy Medical Library (Providence Hospital and Medical Centers), http://www.providence-hospital.org/library/

- **Michigan:** Marquette General Hospital - Consumer Health Library (Marquette General Hospital, Health Information Center), http://www.mgh.org/center.html

- **Michigan:** Patient Education Resouce Center - University of Michigan Cancer Center (University of Michigan Comprehensive Cancer Center, Ann Arbor), http://www.cancer.med.umich.edu/learn/leares.htm

- **Michigan:** Sladen Library & Center for Health Information Resources - Consumer Health Information (Detroit), http://www.henryford.com/body.cfm?id=39330

- **Montana:** Center for Health Information (St. Patrick Hospital and Health Sciences Center, Missoula)

- **National:** Consumer Health Library Directory (Medical Library Association, Consumer and Patient Health Information Section), http://caphis.mlanet.org/directory/index.html

- **National:** National Network of Libraries of Medicine (National Library of Medicine) - provides library services for health professionals in the United States who do not have access to a medical library, http://nnlm.gov/

- **National:** NN/LM List of Libraries Serving the Public (National Network of Libraries of Medicine), http://nnlm.gov/members/

- **Nevada:** Health Science Library, West Charleston Library (Las Vegas-Clark County Library District, Las Vegas), http://www.lvccld.org/special_collections/medical/index.htm

- **New Hampshire:** Dartmouth Biomedical Libraries (Dartmouth College Library, Hanover), http://www.dartmouth.edu/~biomed/resources.htmld/conshealth.htmld/

- **New Jersey:** Consumer Health Library (Rahway Hospital, Rahway), http://www.rahwayhospital.com/library.htm

- **New Jersey:** Dr. Walter Phillips Health Sciences Library (Englewood Hospital and Medical Center, Englewood), http://www.englewoodhospital.com/links/index.htm

- **New Jersey:** Meland Foundation (Englewood Hospital and Medical Center, Englewood), http://www.geocities.com/ResearchTriangle/9360/

- **New York:** Choices in Health Information (New York Public Library) - NLM Consumer Pilot Project participant, http://www.nypl.org/branch/health/links.html

- **New York:** Health Information Center (Upstate Medical University, State University of New York, Syracuse), http://www.upstate.edu/library/hic/

- **New York:** Health Sciences Library (Long Island Jewish Medical Center, New Hyde Park), http://www.lij.edu/library/library.html

- **New York:** ViaHealth Medical Library (Rochester General Hospital), http://www.nyam.org/library/

- **Ohio:** Consumer Health Library (Akron General Medical Center, Medical & Consumer Health Library), http://www.akrongeneral.org/hwlibrary.htm

- **Oklahoma:** The Health Information Center at Saint Francis Hospital (Saint Francis Health System, Tulsa), http://www.sfh-tulsa.com/services/healthinfo.asp

- **Oregon:** Planetree Health Resource Center (Mid-Columbia Medical Center, The Dalles), http://www.mcmc.net/phrc/

- **Pennsylvania:** Community Health Information Library (Milton S. Hershey Medical Center, Hershey), http://www.hmc.psu.edu/commhealth/

- **Pennsylvania:** Community Health Resource Library (Geisinger Medical Center, Danville), http://www.geisinger.edu/education/commlib.shtml

- **Pennsylvania:** HealthInfo Library (Moses Taylor Hospital, Scranton), http://www.mth.org/healthwellness.html

- **Pennsylvania:** Hopwood Library (University of Pittsburgh, Health Sciences Library System, Pittsburgh), http://www.hsls.pitt.edu/guides/chi/hopwood/index_html

- **Pennsylvania:** Koop Community Health Information Center (College of Physicians of Philadelphia), http://www.collphyphil.org/kooppg1.shtml

- **Pennsylvania:** Learning Resources Center - Medical Library (Susquehanna Health System, Williamsport), http://www.shscares.org/services/lrc/index.asp

- **Pennsylvania:** Medical Library (UPMC Health System, Pittsburgh), http://www.upmc.edu/passavant/library.htm

- **Quebec, Canada:** Medical Library (Montreal General Hospital), http://www.mghlib.mcgill.ca/

- **South Dakota:** Rapid City Regional Hospital Medical Library (Rapid City Regional Hospital), **http://www.rcrh.org/Services/Library/Default.asp**

- **Texas:** Houston HealthWays (Houston Academy of Medicine-Texas Medical Center Library), **http://hhw.library.tmc.edu/**

- **Washington:** Community Health Library (Kittitas Valley Community Hospital), **http://www.kvch.com/**

- **Washington:** Southwest Washington Medical Center Library (Southwest Washington Medical Center, Vancouver), **http://www.swmedicalcenter.com/body.cfm?id=72**

ONLINE GLOSSARIES

The Internet provides access to a number of free-to-use medical dictionaries. The National Library of Medicine has compiled the following list of online dictionaries:

- ADAM Medical Encyclopedia (A.D.A.M., Inc.), comprehensive medical reference:
  http://www.nlm.nih.gov/medlineplus/encyclopedia.html

- MedicineNet.com Medical Dictionary (MedicineNet, Inc.):
  http://www.medterms.com/Script/Main/hp.asp

- Merriam-Webster Medical Dictionary (Inteli-Health, Inc.):
  http://www.intelihealth.com/IH/

- Multilingual Glossary of Technical and Popular Medical Terms in Eight European Languages (European Commission) - Danish, Dutch, English, French, German, Italian, Portuguese, and Spanish: **http://allserv.rug.ac.be/~rvdstich/eugloss/welcome.html**

- On-line Medical Dictionary (CancerWEB): **http://cancerweb.ncl.ac.uk/omd/**

- Rare Diseases Terms (Office of Rare Diseases):
  http://ord.aspensys.com/asp/diseases/diseases.asp

- Technology Glossary (National Library of Medicine) - Health Care Technology:
  http://www.nlm.nih.gov/nichsr/ta101/ta10108.htm

Beyond these, MEDLINEplus contains a very patient-friendly encyclopedia covering every aspect of medicine (licensed from A.D.A.M., Inc.). The ADAM Medical Encyclopedia can be accessed at **http://www.nlm.nih.gov/medlineplus/encyclopedia.html**. ADAM is also available on commercial Web sites such as drkoop.com (**http://www.drkoop.com/**) and Web MD (**http://my.webmd.com/adam/asset/adam_disease_articles/a_to_z/a**).

Online Dictionary Directories

The following are additional online directories compiled by the National Library of Medicine, including a number of specialized medical dictionaries:

- Medical Dictionaries: Medical & Biological (World Health Organization):
  http://www.who.int/hlt/virtuallibrary/English/diction.htm#Medical

- MEL-Michigan Electronic Library List of Online Health and Medical Dictionaries (Michigan Electronic Library): **http://mel.lib.mi.us/health/health-dictionaries.html**

- Patient Education: Glossaries (DMOZ Open Directory Project):
  http://dmoz.org/Health/Education/Patient_Education/Glossaries/

- Web of Online Dictionaries (Bucknell University):
  http://www.yourdictionary.com/diction5.html#medicine

ROYAL JELLY DICTIONARY

The definitions below are derived from official public sources, including the National Institutes of Health [NIH] and the European Union [EU].

Abdominal: Having to do with the abdomen, which is the part of the body between the chest and the hips that contains the pancreas, stomach, intestines, liver, gallbladder, and other organs. [NIH]

Adjuvant: A substance which aids another, such as an auxiliary remedy; in immunology, nonspecific stimulator (e.g., BCG vaccine) of the immune response. [EU]

Adrenal Cortex: The outer layer of the adrenal gland. It secretes mineralocorticoids, androgens, and glucocorticoids. [NIH]

Adverse Effect: An unwanted side effect of treatment. [NIH]

Affinity: 1. Inherent likeness or relationship. 2. A special attraction for a specific element, organ, or structure. 3. Chemical affinity; the force that binds atoms in molecules; the tendency of substances to combine by chemical reaction. 4. The strength of noncovalent chemical binding between two substances as measured by the dissociation constant of the complex. 5. In immunology, a thermodynamic expression of the strength of interaction between a single antigen-binding site and a single antigenic determinant (and thus of the stereochemical compatibility between them), most accurately applied to interactions among simple, uniform antigenic determinants such as haptens. Expressed as the association constant (K litres mole -1), which, owing to the heterogeneity of affinities in a population of antibody molecules of a given specificity, actually represents an average value (mean intrinsic association constant). 6. The reciprocal of the dissociation constant. [EU]

Albumin: 1. Any protein that is soluble in water and moderately concentrated salt solutions and is coagulable by heat. 2. Serum albumin; the major plasma protein (approximately 60 per cent of the total), which is responsible for much of the plasma colloidal osmotic pressure and serves as a transport protein carrying large organic anions, such as fatty acids, bilirubin, and many drugs, and also carrying certain hormones, such as cortisol and thyroxine, when their specific binding globulins are saturated. Albumin is synthesized in the liver. Low serum levels occur in protein malnutrition, active inflammation and serious hepatic and renal disease. [EU]

Algorithms: A procedure consisting of a sequence of algebraic formulas and/or logical steps to calculate or determine a given task. [NIH]

Alimentary: Pertaining to food or nutritive material, or to the organs of digestion. [EU]

Alkaline: Having the reactions of an alkali. [EU]

Allergen: An antigenic substance capable of producing immediate-type hypersensitivity (allergy). [EU]

Alopecia: Absence of hair from areas where it is normally present. [NIH]

Alternative medicine: Practices not generally recognized by the medical community as standard or conventional medical approaches and used instead of standard treatments. Alternative medicine includes the taking of dietary supplements, megadose vitamins, and herbal preparations; the drinking of special teas; and practices such as massage therapy, magnet therapy, spiritual healing, and meditation. [NIH]

Ameliorated: A changeable condition which prevents the consequence of a failure or accident from becoming as bad as it otherwise would. [NIH]

Amino Acids: Organic compounds that generally contain an amino (-NH2) and a carboxyl (-COOH) group. Twenty alpha-amino acids are the subunits which are polymerized to form proteins. [NIH]

Amino Acids: Organic compounds that generally contain an amino (-NH2) and a carboxyl (-COOH) group. Twenty alpha-amino acids are the subunits which are polymerized to form proteins. [NIH]

Ampicillin: Semi-synthetic derivative of penicillin that functions as an orally active broad-spectrum antibiotic. [NIH]

Analogous: Resembling or similar in some respects, as in function or appearance, but not in origin or development;. [EU]

Anaphylaxis: An acute hypersensitivity reaction due to exposure to a previously encountered antigen. The reaction may include rapidly progressing urticaria, respiratory distress, vascular collapse, systemic shock, and death. [NIH]

Anemia: A reduction in the number of circulating erythrocytes or in the quantity of hemoglobin. [NIH]

Angelica root: The root of any of a group of herbs called Angelica. It has been used in some cultures to treat certain medical problems, including gastrointestinal problems such as loss of appetite, feelings of fullness, and gas. [NIH]

Anions: Negatively charged atoms, radicals or groups of atoms which travel to the anode or positive pole during electrolysis. [NIH]

Antibacterial: A substance that destroys bacteria or suppresses their growth or reproduction. [EU]

Antibiotic: A drug used to treat infections caused by bacteria and other microorganisms. [NIH]

Antibody: A type of protein made by certain white blood cells in response to a foreign substance (antigen). Each antibody can bind to only a specific antigen. The purpose of this binding is to help destroy the antigen. Antibodies can work in several ways, depending on the nature of the antigen. Some antibodies destroy antigens directly. Others make it easier for white blood cells to destroy the antigen. [NIH]

Antigen: Any substance which is capable, under appropriate conditions, of inducing a specific immune response and of reacting with the products of that response, that is, with specific antibody or specifically sensitized T-lymphocytes, or both. Antigens may be soluble substances, such as toxins and foreign proteins, or particulate, such as bacteria and tissue cells; however, only the portion of the protein or polysaccharide molecule known as the antigenic determinant (q.v.) combines with antibody or a specific receptor on a lymphocyte. Abbreviated Ag. [EU]

Antimicrobial: Killing microorganisms, or suppressing their multiplication or growth. [EU]

Antimycotic: Suppressing the growth of fungi. [EU]

Antiviral: Destroying viruses or suppressing their replication. [EU]

Anxiety: Persistent feeling of dread, apprehension, and impending disaster. [NIH]

Artemisia: A genus of composite herbs and shrubs with strong-smelling foliage. Included in this genus are A. abrotanum (southernwood), A. absinthium (wormwood), and A. maritima (A. pauciflora), from which santonin is derived. A. absinthium oil contains neurotoxic agents (1-thujone and d-isothujone). [NIH]

Arteries: The vessels carrying blood away from the heart. [NIH]

Bacillus: A genus of Bacillaceae that are spore-forming, rod-shaped cells. Most species are saprophytic soil forms with only a few species being pathogenic. [NIH]

Bacteria: Unicellular prokaryotic microorganisms which generally possess rigid cell walls, multiply by cell division, and exhibit three principal forms: round or coccal, rodlike or bacillary, and spiral or spirochetal. [NIH]

Bacteriophage: A virus whose host is a bacterial cell; A virus that exclusively infects bacteria. It generally has a protein coat surrounding the genome (DNA or RNA). One of the coliphages most extensively studied is the lambda phage, which is also one of the most important. [NIH]

Bacterium: Microscopic organism which may have a spherical, rod-like, or spiral unicellular or non-cellular body. Bacteria usually reproduce through asexual processes. [NIH]

Base: In chemistry, the nonacid part of a salt; a substance that combines with acids to form salts; a substance that dissociates to give hydroxide ions in aqueous solutions; a substance whose molecule or ion can combine with a proton (hydrogen ion); a substance capable of donating a pair of electrons (to an acid) for the formation of a coordinate covalent bond. [EU]

Benign: Not cancerous; does not invade nearby tissue or spread to other parts of the body. [NIH]

Bezoar: A ball of food, mucus, vegetable fiber, hair, or other material that cannot be digested in the stomach. Bezoars can cause blockage, ulcers, and bleeding. [NIH]

Bilirubin: A bile pigment that is a degradation product of heme. [NIH]

Biosynthesis: The building up of a chemical compound in the physiologic processes of a living organism. [EU]

Biotechnology: Body of knowledge related to the use of organisms, cells or cell-derived constituents for the purpose of developing products which are technically, scientifically and clinically useful. Alteration of biologic function at the molecular level (i.e., genetic engineering) is a central focus; laboratory methods used include transfection and cloning technologies, sequence and structure analysis algorithms, computer databases, and gene and protein structure function analysis and prediction. [NIH]

Blastocyst: The mammalian embryo in the post-morula stage in which a fluid-filled cavity, enclosed primarily by trophoblast, contains an inner cell mass which becomes the embryonic disc. [NIH]

Blood Coagulation: The process of the interaction of blood coagulation factors that results in an insoluble fibrin clot. [NIH]

Blood pressure: The pressure of blood against the walls of a blood vessel or heart chamber. Unless there is reference to another location, such as the pulmonary artery or one of the heart chambers, it refers to the pressure in the systemic arteries, as measured, for example, in the forearm. [NIH]

Blood vessel: A tube in the body through which blood circulates. Blood vessels include a network of arteries, arterioles, capillaries, venules, and veins. [NIH]

Body Fluids: Liquid components of living organisms. [NIH]

Branch: Most commonly used for branches of nerves, but applied also to other structures. [NIH]

Breakdown: A physical, metal, or nervous collapse. [NIH]

Broad-spectrum: Effective against a wide range of microorganisms; said of an antibiotic. [EU]

Calcium: A basic element found in nearly all organized tissues. It is a member of the alkaline earth family of metals with the atomic symbol Ca, atomic number 20, and atomic weight 40. Calcium is the most abundant mineral in the body and combines with phosphorus to form calcium phosphate in the bones and teeth. It is essential for the normal functioning of nerves and muscles and plays a role in blood coagulation (as factor IV) and in many enzymatic processes. [NIH]

Calcium Sulfate: It exists in an anhydrous form and in various states of hydration: the hemihydrate is plaster of Paris, the dihydrate is gypsum. It is used in building materials, as a desiccant, in dentistry as an impression material, cast, or die, and in medicine for immobilizing casts and as a tablet excipient. [NIH]

Capsules: Hard or soft soluble containers used for the oral administration of medicine. [NIH]

Carbohydrate: An aldehyde or ketone derivative of a polyhydric alcohol, particularly of the pentahydric and hexahydric alcohols. They are so named because the hydrogen and oxygen are usually in the proportion to form water, $(CH2O)n$. The most important carbohydrates are the starches, sugars, celluloses, and gums. They are classified into mono-, di-, tri-, poly- and heterosaccharides. [EU]

Carbon Dioxide: A colorless, odorless gas that can be formed by the body and is necessary for the respiration cycle of plants and animals. [NIH]

Carcinostatic: Pertaining to slowing or stopping the growth of cancer. [NIH]

Cell: The individual unit that makes up all of the tissues of the body. All living things are made up of one or more cells. [NIH]

Cell Division: The fission of a cell. [NIH]

Cellulose: A polysaccharide with glucose units linked as in cellobiose. It is the chief constituent of plant fibers, cotton being the purest natural form of the substance. As a raw material, it forms the basis for many derivatives used in chromatography, ion exchange materials, explosives manufacturing, and pharmaceutical preparations. [NIH]

Central Nervous System: The main information-processing organs of the nervous system, consisting of the brain, spinal cord, and meninges. [NIH]

Central Nervous System Infections: Pathogenic infections of the brain, spinal cord, and meninges. DNA virus infections; RNA virus infections; bacterial infections; mycoplasma infections; Spirochaetales infections; fungal infections; protozoan infections; helminthiasis; and prion diseases may involve the central nervous system as a primary or secondary process. [NIH]

Cheilitis: Inflammation of the lips. It is of various etiologies and degrees of pathology. [NIH]

Chemotherapy: Treatment with anticancer drugs. [NIH]

Chlorophyll: Porphyrin derivatives containing magnesium that act to convert light energy in photosynthetic organisms. [NIH]

Chronic: A disease or condition that persists or progresses over a long period of time. [NIH]

Chronic Fatigue Syndrome: Fatigue caused by the combined effects of different types of prolonged fatigue. [NIH]

Clinical trial: A research study that tests how well new medical treatments or other interventions work in people. Each study is designed to test new methods of screening, prevention, diagnosis, or treatment of a disease. [NIH]

Cloning: The production of a number of genetically identical individuals; in genetic engineering, a process for the efficient replication of a great number of identical DNA molecules. [NIH]

Codons: Any triplet of nucleotides (coding unit) in DNA or RNA (if RNA is the carrier of primary genetic information as in some viruses) that codes for particular amino acid or signals the beginning or end of the message. [NIH]

Colitis: Inflammation of the colon. [NIH]

Collagen: A polypeptide substance comprising about one third of the total protein in mammalian organisms. It is the main constituent of skin, connective tissue, and the organic substance of bones and teeth. Different forms of collagen are produced in the body but all consist of three alpha-polypeptide chains arranged in a triple helix. Collagen is differentiated from other fibrous proteins, such as elastin, by the content of proline, hydroxyproline, and hydroxylysine; by the absence of tryptophan; and particularly by the high content of polar groups which are responsible for its swelling properties. [NIH]

Collapse: 1. A state of extreme prostration and depression, with failure of circulation. 2. Abnormal falling in of the walls of any part of organ. [EU]

Colloidal: Of the nature of a colloid. [EU]

Complement: A term originally used to refer to the heat-labile factor in serum that causes immune cytolysis, the lysis of antibody-coated cells, and now referring to the entire functionally related system comprising at least 20 distinct serum proteins that is the effector not only of immune cytolysis but also of other biologic functions. Complement activation occurs by two different sequences, the classic and alternative pathways. The proteins of the classic pathway are termed 'components of complement' and are designated by the symbols C1 through C9. C1 is a calcium-dependent complex of three distinct proteins C1q, C1r and C1s. The proteins of the alternative pathway (collectively referred to as the properdin system) and complement regulatory proteins are known by semisystematic or trivial names. Fragments resulting from proteolytic cleavage of complement proteins are designated with lower-case letter suffixes, e.g., C3a. Inactivated fragments may be designated with the suffix 'i', e.g. C3bi. Activated components or complexes with biological activity are designated by a bar over the symbol e.g. C1 or C4b,2a. The classic pathway is activated by the binding of C1 to classic pathway activators, primarily antigen-antibody complexes containing IgM, IgG1, IgG3; C1q binds to a single IgM molecule or two adjacent IgG molecules. The alternative pathway can be activated by IgA immune complexes and also by nonimmunologic materials including bacterial endotoxins, microbial polysaccharides, and cell walls. Activation of the classic pathway triggers an enzymatic cascade involving C1, C4, C2 and C3; activation of the alternative pathway triggers a cascade involving C3 and factors B, D and P. Both result in the cleavage of C5 and the formation of the membrane attack complex. Complement activation also results in the formation of many biologically active complement fragments that act as anaphylatoxins, opsonins, or chemotactic factors. [EU]

Complementary and alternative medicine: CAM. Forms of treatment that are used in addition to (complementary) or instead of (alternative) standard treatments. These practices are not considered standard medical approaches. CAM includes dietary supplements, megadose vitamins, herbal preparations, special teas, massage therapy, magnet therapy, spiritual healing, and meditation. [NIH]

Complementary medicine: Practices not generally recognized by the medical community as standard or conventional medical approaches and used to enhance or complement the standard treatments. Complementary medicine includes the taking of dietary supplements, megadose vitamins, and herbal preparations; the drinking of special teas; and practices such as massage therapy, magnet therapy, spiritual healing, and meditation. [NIH]

Computational Biology: A field of biology concerned with the development of techniques for the collection and manipulation of biological data, and the use of such data to make biological discoveries or predictions. This field encompasses all computational methods and theories applicable to molecular biology and areas of computer-based techniques for solving biological problems including manipulation of models and datasets. [NIH]

Connective Tissue: Tissue that supports and binds other tissues. It consists of connective tissue cells embedded in a large amount of extracellular matrix. [NIH]

Connective Tissue: Tissue that supports and binds other tissues. It consists of connective tissue cells embedded in a large amount of extracellular matrix. [NIH]

Connective Tissue Cells: A group of cells that includes fibroblasts, cartilage cells, adipocytes, smooth muscle cells, and bone cells. [NIH]

Consumption: Pulmonary tuberculosis. [NIH]

Contraindications: Any factor or sign that it is unwise to pursue a certain kind of action or treatment, e. g. giving a general anesthetic to a person with pneumonia. [NIH]

Coronary: Encircling in the manner of a crown; a term applied to vessels; nerves, ligaments, etc. The term usually denotes the arteries that supply the heart muscle and, by extension, a pathologic involvement of them. [EU]

Coronary Thrombosis: Presence of a thrombus in a coronary artery, often causing a myocardial infarction. [NIH]

Corpus: The body of the uterus. [NIH]

Corpus Luteum: The yellow glandular mass formed in the ovary by an ovarian follicle that has ruptured and discharged its ovum. [NIH]

Cortisol: A steroid hormone secreted by the adrenal cortex as part of the body's response to stress. [NIH]

Cranial: Pertaining to the cranium, or to the anterior (in animals) or superior (in humans) end of the body. [EU]

Craniocerebral Trauma: Traumatic injuries involving the cranium and intracranial structures (i.e., brain; cranial nerves; meninges; and other structures). Injuries may be classified by whether or not the skull is penetrated (i.e., penetrating vs. nonpenetrating) or whether there is an associated hemorrhage. [NIH]

Crystallization: The formation of crystals; conversion to a crystalline form. [EU]

Curative: Tending to overcome disease and promote recovery. [EU]

Databases, Bibliographic: Extensive collections, reputedly complete, of references and citations to books, articles, publications, etc., generally on a single subject or specialized subject area. Databases can operate through automated files, libraries, or computer disks. The concept should be differentiated from factual databases which is used for collections of data and facts apart from bibliographic references to them. [NIH]

Decidua: The epithelial lining of the endometrium that is formed before the fertilized ovum reaches the uterus. The fertilized ovum embeds in the decidua. If the ovum is not fertilized, the decidua is shed during menstruation. [NIH]

Dermatitis: Any inflammation of the skin. [NIH]

Diagnostic procedure: A method used to identify a disease. [NIH]

Digestion: The process of breakdown of food for metabolism and use by the body. [NIH]

Diploid: Having two sets of chromosomes. [NIH]

Direct: 1. Straight; in a straight line. 2. Performed immediately and without the intervention of subsidiary means. [EU]

Dross: Residue remaining in an opium pipe which has been smoked; contains 50 % of the morphine present in the original drug. [NIH]

Duct: A tube through which body fluids pass. [NIH]

Dysphoria: Disquiet; restlessness; malaise. [EU]

Edema: Excessive amount of watery fluid accumulated in the intercellular spaces, most commonly present in subcutaneous tissue. [NIH]

Electrolyte: A substance that dissociates into ions when fused or in solution, and thus becomes capable of conducting electricity; an ionic solute. [EU]

Embryo: The prenatal stage of mammalian development characterized by rapid morphological changes and the differentiation of basic structures. [NIH]

Endometrium: The layer of tissue that lines the uterus. [NIH]

Environmental Health: The science of controlling or modifying those conditions, influences, or forces surrounding man which relate to promoting, establishing, and maintaining health. [NIH]

Enzymatic: Phase where enzyme cuts the precursor protein. [NIH]

Enzyme: A protein that speeds up chemical reactions in the body. [NIH]

Epithelial: Refers to the cells that line the internal and external surfaces of the body. [NIH]

Epithelial Cells: Cells that line the inner and outer surfaces of the body. [NIH]

Erythritol: A four-carbon sugar that is found in algae, fungi, and lichens. It is twice as sweet as sucrose and can be used as a coronary vasodilator. [NIH]

Erythrocytes: Red blood cells. Mature erythrocytes are non-nucleated, biconcave disks containing hemoglobin whose function is to transport oxygen. [NIH]

Estrogen: One of the two female sex hormones. [NIH]

Ethanol: A clear, colorless liquid rapidly absorbed from the gastrointestinal tract and distributed throughout the body. It has bactericidal activity and is used often as a topical disinfectant. It is widely used as a solvent and preservative in pharmaceutical preparations as well as serving as the primary ingredient in alcoholic beverages. [NIH]

Excipient: Any more or less inert substance added to a prescription in order to confer a suitable consistency or form to the drug; a vehicle. [EU]

Exocrine: Secreting outwardly, via a duct. [EU]

Extracellular: Outside a cell or cells. [EU]

Extracellular Matrix: A meshwork-like substance found within the extracellular space and in association with the basement membrane of the cell surface. It promotes cellular proliferation and provides a supporting structure to which cells or cell lysates in culture dishes adhere. [NIH]

Extraction: The process or act of pulling or drawing out. [EU]

Family Planning: Programs or services designed to assist the family in controlling reproduction by either improving or diminishing fertility. [NIH]

Fat: Total lipids including phospholipids. [NIH]

Fatigue: The state of weariness following a period of exertion, mental or physical, characterized by a decreased capacity for work and reduced efficiency to respond to stimuli. [NIH]

Fatty acids: A major component of fats that are used by the body for energy and tissue development. [NIH]

Fermentation: An enzyme-induced chemical change in organic compounds that takes place in the absence of oxygen. The change usually results in the production of ethanol or lactic acid, and the production of energy. [NIH]

Fetus: The developing offspring from 7 to 8 weeks after conception until birth. [NIH]

Fixation: 1. The act or operation of holding, suturing, or fastening in a fixed position. 2. The condition of being held in a fixed position. 3. In psychiatry, a term with two related but distinct meanings : (1) arrest of development at a particular stage, which like regression (return to an earlier stage), if temporary is a normal reaction to setbacks and difficulties but if protracted or frequent is a cause of developmental failures and emotional problems, and (2) a close and suffocating attachment to another person, especially a childhood figure, such as one's mother or father. Both meanings are derived from psychoanalytic theory and refer to 'fixation' of libidinal energy either in a specific erogenous zone, hence fixation at the oral, anal, or phallic stage, or in a specific object, hence mother or father fixation. 4. The use of a fixative (q.v.) to preserve histological or cytological specimens. 5. In chemistry, the process whereby a substance is removed from the gaseous or solution phase and localized, as in carbon dioxide fixation or nitrogen fixation. 6. In ophthalmology, direction of the gaze so that the visual image of the object falls on the fovea centralis. 7. In film processing, the chemical removal of all undeveloped salts of the film emulsion, leaving only the developed silver to form a permanent image. [EU]

Flatus: Gas passed through the rectum. [NIH]

Flushing: A transient reddening of the face that may be due to fever, certain drugs, exertion, stress, or a disease process. [NIH]

Forearm: The part between the elbow and the wrist. [NIH]

Fungi: A kingdom of eukaryotic, heterotrophic organisms that live as saprobes or parasites, including mushrooms, yeasts, smuts, molds, etc. They reproduce either sexually or asexually, and have life cycles that range from simple to complex. Filamentous fungi refer to those that grow as multicelluar colonies (mushrooms and molds). [NIH]

Fungus: A general term used to denote a group of eukaryotic protists, including mushrooms, yeasts, rusts, moulds, smuts, etc., which are characterized by the absence of chlorophyll and by the presence of a rigid cell wall composed of chitin, mannans, and sometimes cellulose. They are usually of simple morphological form or show some reversible cellular specialization, such as the formation of pseudoparenchymatous tissue in the fruiting body of a mushroom. The dimorphic fungi grow, according to environmental conditions, as moulds or yeasts. [EU]

Gallbladder: The pear-shaped organ that sits below the liver. Bile is concentrated and stored in the gallbladder. [NIH]

Gas: Air that comes from normal breakdown of food. The gases are passed out of the body through the rectum (flatus) or the mouth (burp). [NIH]

Gastrin: A hormone released after eating. Gastrin causes the stomach to produce more acid. [NIH]

Gastrointestinal: Refers to the stomach and intestines. [NIH]

Gelatin: A product formed from skin, white connective tissue, or bone collagen. It is used as a protein food adjuvant, plasma substitute, hemostatic, suspending agent in pharmaceutical preparations, and in the manufacturing of capsules and suppositories. [NIH]

Gene: The functional and physical unit of heredity passed from parent to offspring. Genes are pieces of DNA, and most genes contain the information for making a specific protein. [NIH]

Gestation: The period of development of the young in viviparous animals, from the time of fertilization of the ovum until birth. [EU]

Ginger: Deciduous plant rich in volatile oil (oils, volatile). It is used as a flavoring agent and has many other uses both internally and topically. [NIH]

Ginseng: An araliaceous genus of plants that contains a number of pharmacologically active agents used as stimulants, sedatives, and tonics, especially in traditional medicine. [NIH]

Gland: An organ that produces and releases one or more substances for use in the body. Some glands produce fluids that affect tissues or organs. Others produce hormones or participate in blood production. [NIH]

Glycine: A non-essential amino acid. It is found primarily in gelatin and silk fibroin and used therapeutically as a nutrient. It is also a fast inhibitory neurotransmitter. [NIH]

Glycoprotein: A protein that has sugar molecules attached to it. [NIH]

Governing Board: The group in which legal authority is vested for the control of health-related institutions and organizations. [NIH]

Growth: The progressive development of a living being or part of an organism from its earliest stage to maturity. [NIH]

Haploid: An organism with one basic chromosome set, symbolized by n; the normal condition of gametes in diploids. [NIH]

Headache: Pain in the cranial region that may occur as an isolated and benign symptom or as a manifestation of a wide variety of conditions including subarachnoid hemorrhage; craniocerebral trauma; central nervous system infections; intracranial hypertension; and other disorders. In general, recurrent headaches that are not associated with a primary disease process are referred to as headache disorders (e.g., migraine). [NIH]

Headache Disorders: Common conditions characterized by persistent or recurrent headaches. Headache syndrome classification systems may be based on etiology (e.g., vascular headache, post-traumatic headaches, etc.), temporal pattern (e.g., cluster headache, paroxysmal hemicrania, etc.), and precipitating factors (e.g., cough headache). [NIH]

Hemoglobin: One of the fractions of glycosylated hemoglobin A1c. Glycosylated hemoglobin is formed when linkages of glucose and related monosaccharides bind to hemoglobin A and its concentration represents the average blood glucose level over the previous several weeks. HbA1c levels are used as a measure of long-term control of plasma glucose (normal, 4 to 6 percent). In controlled diabetes mellitus, the concentration of glycosylated hemoglobin A is within the normal range, but in uncontrolled cases the level may be 3 to 4 times the normal conentration. Generally, complications are substantially lower among patients with Hb levels of 7 percent or less than in patients with HbA1c levels of 9 percent or more. [NIH]

Hemorrhage: Bleeding or escape of blood from a vessel. [NIH]

Hepatic: Refers to the liver. [NIH]

Hepatocytes: The main structural component of the liver. They are specialized epithelial cells that are organized into interconnected plates called lobules. [NIH]

Heredity: 1. The genetic transmission of a particular quality or trait from parent to offspring. 2. The genetic constitution of an individual. [EU]

Homologous: Corresponding in structure, position, origin, etc., as (a) the feathers of a bird and the scales of a fish, (b) antigen and its specific antibody, (c) allelic chromosomes. [EU]

Hormonal: Pertaining to or of the nature of a hormone. [EU]

Hormone: A substance in the body that regulates certain organs. Hormones such as gastrin help in breaking down food. Some hormones come from cells in the stomach and small intestine. [NIH]

Hybrid: Cross fertilization between two varieties or, more usually, two species of vines, see also crossing. [NIH]

Hydration: Combining with water. [NIH]

Hydrogen: The first chemical element in the periodic table. It has the atomic symbol H, atomic number 1, and atomic weight 1. It exists, under normal conditions, as a colorless, odorless, tasteless, diatomic gas. Hydrogen ions are protons. Besides the common H1 isotope, hydrogen exists as the stable isotope deuterium and the unstable, radioactive isotope tritium. [NIH]

Hypersensitivity: Altered reactivity to an antigen, which can result in pathologic reactions upon subsequent exposure to that particular antigen. [NIH]

Hypertension: Persistently high arterial blood pressure. Currently accepted threshold levels are 140 mm Hg systolic and 90 mm Hg diastolic pressure. [NIH]

Id: The part of the personality structure which harbors the unconscious instinctive desires and strivings of the individual. [NIH]

Immune response: The activity of the immune system against foreign substances (antigens). [NIH]

Immune system: The organs, cells, and molecules responsible for the recognition and disposal of foreign ("non-self") material which enters the body. [NIH]

Immunization: Deliberate stimulation of the host's immune response. Active immunization involves administration of antigens or immunologic adjuvants. Passive immunization involves administration of immune sera or lymphocytes or their extracts (e.g., transfer factor, immune RNA) or transplantation of immunocompetent cell producing tissue (thymus or bone marrow). [NIH]

Immunologic: The ability of the antibody-forming system to recall a previous experience with an antigen and to respond to a second exposure with the prompt production of large amounts of antibody. [NIH]

Immunomodulator: New type of drugs mainly using biotechnological methods. Treatment of cancer. [NIH]

Indicative: That indicates; that points out more or less exactly; that reveals fairly clearly. [EU]

Infarction: A pathological process consisting of a sudden insufficient blood supply to an area, which results in necrosis of that area. It is usually caused by a thrombus, an embolus, or a vascular torsion. [NIH]

Infection: 1. Invasion and multiplication of microorganisms in body tissues, which may be clinically unapparent or result in local cellular injury due to competitive metabolism, toxins, intracellular replication, or antigen-antibody response. The infection may remain localized, subclinical, and temporary if the body's defensive mechanisms are effective. A local infection may persist and spread by extension to become an acute, subacute, or chronic clinical infection or disease state. A local infection may also become systemic when the microorganisms gain access to the lymphatic or vascular system. 2. An infectious disease. [EU]

Infertility: The diminished or absent ability to conceive or produce an offspring while sterility is the complete inability to conceive or produce an offspring. [NIH]

Inflammation: A pathological process characterized by injury or destruction of tissues caused by a variety of cytologic and chemical reactions. It is usually manifested by typical signs of pain, heat, redness, swelling, and loss of function. [NIH]

Ingestion: Taking into the body by mouth [NIH]

Inhalation: The drawing of air or other substances into the lungs. [EU]

Inlay: In dentistry, a filling first made to correspond with the form of a dental cavity and then cemented into the cavity. [NIH]

Inorganic: Pertaining to substances not of organic origin. [EU]

Intestines: The section of the alimentary canal from the stomach to the anus. It includes the large intestine and small intestine. [NIH]

Intracellular: Inside a cell. [NIH]

Introns: Non-coding, intervening sequences of DNA that are transcribed, but are removed from within the primary gene transcript and rapidly degraded during maturation of messenger RNA. Most genes in the nuclei of eukaryotes contain introns, as do mitochondrial and chloroplast genes. [NIH]

Kb: A measure of the length of DNA fragments, 1 Kb = 1000 base pairs. The largest DNA fragments are up to 50 kilobases long. [NIH]

Larva: Wormlike or grublike stage, following the egg in the life cycle of insects, worms, and other metamorphosing animals. [NIH]

Library Services: Services offered to the library user. They include reference and circulation. [NIH]

Lichens: Any of a group of plants formed by a mutual combination of an alga and a fungus. [NIH]

Life cycle: The successive stages through which an organism passes from fertilized ovum or spore to the fertilized ovum or spore of the next generation. [NIH]

Lip: Either of the two fleshy, full-blooded margins of the mouth. [NIH]

Liver: A large, glandular organ located in the upper abdomen. The liver cleanses the blood and aids in digestion by secreting bile. [NIH]

Localized: Cancer which has not metastasized yet. [NIH]

Locomotion: Movement or the ability to move from one place or another. It can refer to humans, vertebrate or invertebrate animals, and microorganisms. [NIH]

Lymphatic: The tissues and organs, including the bone marrow, spleen, thymus, and lymph nodes, that produce and store cells that fight infection and disease. [NIH]

Lymphocytic: Referring to lymphocytes, a type of white blood cell. [NIH]

Macrophage: A type of white blood cell that surrounds and kills microorganisms, removes dead cells, and stimulates the action of other immune system cells. [NIH]

Malaise: A vague feeling of bodily discomfort. [EU]

Malnutrition: A condition caused by not eating enough food or not eating a balanced diet. [NIH]

Mannans: Polysaccharides consisting of mannose units. [NIH]

Medicament: A medicinal substance or agent. [EU]

MEDLINE: An online database of MEDLARS, the computerized bibliographic Medical Literature Analysis and Retrieval System of the National Library of Medicine. [NIH]

Menstrual Cycle: The period of the regularly recurring physiologic changes in the endometrium occurring during the reproductive period in human females and some primates and culminating in partial sloughing of the endometrium (menstruation). [NIH]

Menstruation: The normal physiologic discharge through the vagina of blood and mucosal tissues from the nonpregnant uterus. [NIH]

Metamorphosis: The ontogeny of insects, i. e. the series of changes undergone from egg, through larva and pupa, or through nymph, to adult. [NIH]

MI: Myocardial infarction. Gross necrosis of the myocardium as a result of interruption of the blood supply to the area; it is almost always caused by atherosclerosis of the coronary arteries, upon which coronary thrombosis is usually superimposed. [NIH]

Mitosis: A method of indirect cell division by means of which the two daughter nuclei normally receive identical complements of the number of chromosomes of the somatic cells of the species. [NIH]

Mitotic: Cell resulting from mitosis. [NIH]

Molecular: Of, pertaining to, or composed of molecules : a very small mass of matter. [EU]

Molecule: A chemical made up of two or more atoms. The atoms in a molecule can be the same (an oxygen molecule has two oxygen atoms) or different (a water molecule has two hydrogen atoms and one oxygen atom). Biological molecules, such as proteins and DNA, can be made up of many thousands of atoms. [NIH]

Morphological: Relating to the configuration or the structure of live organs. [NIH]

Mucus: The viscous secretion of mucous membranes. It contains mucin, white blood cells, water, inorganic salts, and exfoliated cells. [NIH]

Myocardium: The muscle tissue of the heart composed of striated, involuntary muscle known as cardiac muscle. [NIH]

Necrosis: A pathological process caused by the progressive degradative action of enzymes that is generally associated with severe cellular trauma. It is characterized by mitochondrial swelling, nuclear flocculation, uncontrolled cell lysis, and ultimately cell death. [NIH]

Need: A state of tension or dissatisfaction felt by an individual that impels him to action toward a goal he believes will satisfy the impulse. [NIH]

Neurotoxic: Poisonous or destructive to nerve tissue. [EU]

Nutritive Value: An indication of the contribution of a food to the nutrient content of the diet. This value depends on the quantity of a food which is digested and absorbed and the amounts of the essential nutrients (protein, fat, carbohydrate, minerals, vitamins) which it contains. This value can be affected by soil and growing conditions, handling and storage, and processing. [NIH]

Nymph: The immature stage in the life cycle of those orders of insects characterized by gradual metamorphosis, in which the young resemble the imago in general form of body, including compound eyes and external wings; also the 8-legged stage of mites and ticks that follows the first moult. [NIH]

Osmotic: Pertaining to or of the nature of osmosis (= the passage of pure solvent from a solution of lesser to one of greater solute concentration when the two solutions are separated by a membrane which selectively prevents the passage of solute molecules, but is permeable to the solvent). [EU]

Ovary: Either of the paired glands in the female that produce the female germ cells and secrete some of the female sex hormones. [NIH]

Ovum: A female germ cell extruded from the ovary at ovulation. [NIH]

Pancreas: A mixed exocrine and endocrine gland situated transversely across the posterior abdominal wall in the epigastric and hypochondriac regions. The endocrine portion is comprised of the Islets of Langerhans, while the exocrine portion is a compound acinar gland that secretes digestive enzymes. [NIH]

Particle: A tiny mass of material. [EU]

Pathologic: 1. Indicative of or caused by a morbid condition. 2. Pertaining to pathology (= branch of medicine that treats the essential nature of the disease, especially the structural and functional changes in tissues and organs of the body caused by the disease). [EU]

Penicillin: An antibiotic drug used to treat infection. [NIH]

Peptide: Any compound consisting of two or more amino acids, the building blocks of proteins. Peptides are combined to make proteins. [NIH]

Pharmaceutical Preparations: Drugs intended for human or veterinary use, presented in their finished dosage form. Included here are materials used in the preparation and/or formulation of the finished dosage form. [NIH]

Pharmacologic: Pertaining to pharmacology or to the properties and reactions of drugs. [EU]

Phospholipids: Lipids containing one or more phosphate groups, particularly those derived from either glycerol (phosphoglycerides; glycerophospholipids) or sphingosine (sphingolipids). They are polar lipids that are of great importance for the structure and function of cell membranes and are the most abundant of membrane lipids, although not stored in large amounts in the system. [NIH]

Phosphorus: A non-metallic element that is found in the blood, muscles, nevers, bones, and teeth, and is a component of adenosine triphosphate (ATP; the primary energy source for the body's cells.) [NIH]

Physiologic: Having to do with the functions of the body. When used in the phrase "physiologic age," it refers to an age assigned by general health, as opposed to calendar age. [NIH]

Placenta: A highly vascular fetal organ through which the fetus absorbs oxygen and other nutrients and excretes carbon dioxide and other wastes. It begins to form about the eighth day of gestation when the blastocyst adheres to the decidua. [NIH]

Plants: Multicellular, eukaryotic life forms of the kingdom Plantae. They are characterized by a mainly photosynthetic mode of nutrition; essentially unlimited growth at localized regions of cell divisions (meristems); cellulose within cells providing rigidity; the absence of organs of locomotion; absense of nervous and sensory systems; and an alteration of haploid and diploid generations. [NIH]

Plasma: The clear, yellowish, fluid part of the blood that carries the blood cells. The proteins that form blood clots are in plasma. [NIH]

Plasma protein: One of the hundreds of different proteins present in blood plasma, including carrier proteins (such albumin, transferrin, and haptoglobin), fibrinogen and other coagulation factors, complement components, immunoglobulins, enzyme inhibitors, precursors of substances such as angiotension and bradykinin, and many other types of proteins. [EU]

Pollen: The male fertilizing element of flowering plants analogous to sperm in animals. It is released from the anthers as yellow dust, to be carried by insect or other vectors, including wind, to the ovary (stigma) of other flowers to produce the embryo enclosed by the seed. The pollens of many plants are allergenic. [NIH]

Polymorphic: Occurring in several or many forms; appearing in different forms at different stages of development. [EU]

Practice Guidelines: Directions or principles presenting current or future rules of policy for the health care practitioner to assist him in patient care decisions regarding diagnosis, therapy, or related clinical circumstances. The guidelines may be developed by government agencies at any level, institutions, professional societies, governing boards, or by the convening of expert panels. The guidelines form a basis for the evaluation of all aspects of health care and delivery. [NIH]

Precursor: Something that precedes. In biological processes, a substance from which another, usually more active or mature substance is formed. In clinical medicine, a sign or symptom that heralds another. [EU]

Progesterone: Pregn-4-ene-3,20-dione. The principal progestational hormone of the body, secreted by the corpus luteum, adrenal cortex, and placenta. Its chief function is to prepare the uterus for the reception and development of the fertilized ovum. It acts as an antiovulatory agent when administered on days 5-25 of the menstrual cycle. [NIH]

Progressive: Advancing; going forward; going from bad to worse; increasing in scope or severity. [EU]

Propolis: Resinous substance obtained from beehives; contains many different substances which may have antimicrobial or antimycotic activity topically; its extracts are called propolis resin or balsam. Synonyms: bee bread; hive dross; bee glue. [NIH]

Protein C: A vitamin-K dependent zymogen present in the blood, which, upon activation by thrombin and thrombomodulin exerts anticoagulant properties by inactivating factors Va and VIIIa at the rate-limiting steps of thrombin formation. [NIH]

Protein S: The vitamin K-dependent cofactor of activated protein C. Together with protein C, it inhibits the action of factors VIIIa and Va. A deficiency in protein S can lead to recurrent venous and arterial thrombosis. [NIH]

Proteins: Polymers of amino acids linked by peptide bonds. The specific sequence of amino acids determines the shape and function of the protein. [NIH]

Public Policy: A course or method of action selected, usually by a government, from among alternatives to guide and determine present and future decisions. [NIH]

Pulmonary: Relating to the lungs. [NIH]

Pulmonary Artery: The short wide vessel arising from the conus arteriosus of the right ventricle and conveying unaerated blood to the lungs. [NIH]

Pupa: An inactive stage between the larval and adult stages in the life cycle of insects. [NIH]

Purines: A series of heterocyclic compounds that are variously substituted in nature and are known also as purine bases. They include adenine and guanine, constituents of nucleic acids, as well as many alkaloids such as caffeine and theophylline. Uric acid is the metabolic end product of purine metabolism. [NIH]

Recombinant: A cell or an individual with a new combination of genes not found together in either parent; usually applied to linked genes. [EU]

Rectum: The last 8 to 10 inches of the large intestine. [NIH]

Refer: To send or direct for treatment, aid, information, de decision. [NIH]

Regimen: A treatment plan that specifies the dosage, the schedule, and the duration of treatment. [NIH]

Restoration: Broad term applied to any inlay, crown, bridge or complete denture which restores or replaces loss of teeth or oral tissues. [NIH]

Rigidity: Stiffness or inflexibility, chiefly that which is abnormal or morbid; rigor. [EU]

Rod: A reception for vision, located in the retina. [NIH]

Screening: Checking for disease when there are no symptoms. [NIH]

Secretion: 1. The process of elaborating a specific product as a result of the activity of a gland; this activity may range from separating a specific substance of the blood to the elaboration of a new chemical substance. 2. Any substance produced by secretion. [EU]

Sensitization: 1. Administration of antigen to induce a primary immune response; priming; immunization. 2. Exposure to allergen that results in the development of hypersensitivity. 3. The coating of erythrocytes with antibody so that they are subject to lysis by complement in the presence of homologous antigen, the first stage of a complement fixation test. [EU]

Serine: A non-essential amino acid occurring in natural form as the L-isomer. It is synthesized from glycine or threonine. It is involved in the biosynthesis of purines, pyrimidines, and other amino acids. [NIH]

Serum: The clear liquid part of the blood that remains after blood cells and clotting proteins have been removed. [NIH]

Shock: The general bodily disturbance following a severe injury; an emotional or moral upset occasioned by some disturbing or unexpected experience; disruption of the circulation, which can upset all body functions: sometimes referred to as circulatory shock. [NIH]

Side effect: A consequence other than the one(s) for which an agent or measure is used, as the adverse effects produced by a drug, especially on a tissue or organ system other than the one sought to be benefited by its administration. [EU]

Small intestine: The part of the digestive tract that is located between the stomach and the large intestine. [NIH]

Sodium: An element that is a member of the alkali group of metals. It has the atomic symbol Na, atomic number 11, and atomic weight 23. With a valence of 1, it has a strong affinity for oxygen and other nonmetallic elements. Sodium provides the chief cation of the extracellular body fluids. Its salts are the most widely used in medicine. (From Dorland, 27th ed) Physiologically the sodium ion plays a major role in blood pressure regulation, maintenance of fluid volume, and electrolyte balance. [NIH]

Specialist: In medicine, one who concentrates on 1 special branch of medical science. [NIH]

Species: A taxonomic category subordinate to a genus (or subgenus) and superior to a subspecies or variety, composed of individuals possessing common characters distinguishing them from other categories of individuals of the same taxonomic level. In taxonomic nomenclature, species are designated by the genus name followed by a Latin or Latinized adjective or noun. [EU]

Sperm: The fecundating fluid of the male. [NIH]

Sterile: Unable to produce children. [NIH]

Sterility: 1. The inability to produce offspring, i.e., the inability to conceive (female s.) or to induce conception (male s.). 2. The state of being aseptic, or free from microorganisms. [EU]

Stimulant: 1. Producing stimulation; especially producing stimulation by causing tension on muscle fibre through the nervous tissue. 2. An agent or remedy that produces stimulation. [EU]

Stomach: An organ of digestion situated in the left upper quadrant of the abdomen between the termination of the esophagus and the beginning of the duodenum. [NIH]

Stress: Forcibly exerted influence; pressure. Any condition or situation that causes strain or tension. Stress may be either physical or psychologic, or both. [NIH]

Subacute: Somewhat acute; between acute and chronic. [EU]

Subarachnoid: Situated or occurring between the arachnoid and the pia mater. [EU]

Subclinical: Without clinical manifestations; said of the early stage(s) of an infection or other disease or abnormality before symptoms and signs become apparent or detectable by clinical examination or laboratory tests, or of a very mild form of an infection or other disease or abnormality. [EU]

Subcutaneous: Beneath the skin. [NIH]

Substance P: An eleven-amino acid neurotransmitter that appears in both the central and peripheral nervous systems. It is involved in transmission of pain, causes rapid contractions of the gastrointestinal smooth muscle, and modulates inflammatory and immune responses.

[NIH]

Suppositories: A small cone-shaped medicament having cocoa butter or gelatin at its basis and usually intended for the treatment of local conditions in the rectum. [NIH]

Synergistic: Acting together; enhancing the effect of another force or agent. [EU]

Systemic: Affecting the entire body. [NIH]

Threonine: An essential amino acid occurring naturally in the L-form, which is the active form. It is found in eggs, milk, gelatin, and other proteins. [NIH]

Thyroxine: An amino acid of the thyroid gland which exerts a stimulating effect on thyroid metabolism. [NIH]

Tissue: A group or layer of cells that are alike in type and work together to perform a specific function. [NIH]

Tonic: 1. Producing and restoring the normal tone. 2. Characterized by continuous tension. 3. A term formerly used for a class of medicinal preparations believed to have the power of restoring normal tone to tissue. [EU]

Tonicity: The normal state of muscular tension. [NIH]

Topical: On the surface of the body. [NIH]

Toxic: Having to do with poison or something harmful to the body. Toxic substances usually cause unwanted side effects. [NIH]

Toxicology: The science concerned with the detection, chemical composition, and pharmacologic action of toxic substances or poisons and the treatment and prevention of toxic manifestations. [NIH]

Toxins: Specific, characterizable, poisonous chemicals, often proteins, with specific biological properties, including immunogenicity, produced by microbes, higher plants, or animals. [NIH]

Trace element: Substance or element essential to plant or animal life, but present in extremely small amounts. [NIH]

Transduction: The transfer of genes from one cell to another by means of a viral (in the case of bacteria, a bacteriophage) vector or a vector which is similar to a virus particle (pseudovirion). [NIH]

Transfection: The uptake of naked or purified DNA into cells, usually eukaryotic. It is analogous to bacterial transformation. [NIH]

Tuberculosis: Any of the infectious diseases of man and other animals caused by species of Mycobacterium. [NIH]

Unconscious: Experience which was once conscious, but was subsequently rejected, as the "personal unconscious". [NIH]

Urticaria: A vascular reaction of the skin characterized by erythema and wheal formation due to localized increase of vascular permeability. The causative mechanism may be allergy, infection, or stress. [NIH]

Uterus: The small, hollow, pear-shaped organ in a woman's pelvis. This is the organ in which a fetus develops. Also called the womb. [NIH]

Valine: A branched-chain essential amino acid that has stimulant activity. It promotes muscle growth and tissue repair. It is a precursor in the penicillin biosynthetic pathway. [NIH]

Vascular: Pertaining to blood vessels or indicative of a copious blood supply. [EU]

Vasodilator: An agent that widens blood vessels. [NIH]

Vector: Plasmid or other self-replicating DNA molecule that transfers DNA between cells in nature or in recombinant DNA technology. [NIH]

Veterinary Medicine: The medical science concerned with the prevention, diagnosis, and treatment of diseases in animals. [NIH]

Viral: Pertaining to, caused by, or of the nature of virus. [EU]

Virus: Submicroscopic organism that causes infectious disease. In cancer therapy, some viruses may be made into vaccines that help the body build an immune response to, and kill, tumor cells. [NIH]

Vitellogenin: A serum and yolk protein which has been characterized as a calcium-binding glycolipophosphoprotein. It is induced by estrogen or juvenile hormone and is essential for yolk formation in various insect species. [NIH]

White blood cell: A type of cell in the immune system that helps the body fight infection and disease. White blood cells include lymphocytes, granulocytes, macrophages, and others. [NIH]

Wound Healing: Restoration of integrity to traumatized tissue. [NIH]

Yeasts: A general term for single-celled rounded fungi that reproduce by budding. Brewers' and bakers' yeasts are Saccharomyces cerevisiae; therapeutic dried yeast is dried yeast. [NIH]

INDEX

Printed in the United States
19319LVS00002B/349

9 780597 842979